Chair Yoga Essentials

Easy Steps to Health and Flexibility

by
Mike Ezekiel

Chair Yoga Essentials

Easy Steps to Health and Flexibility

Table of Contents

Introduction

Welcome to a journey that intertwines the grace of yoga with the practicality of daily life, making wellness accessible right from your chair. The pursuit of health and flexibility need not be restricted to those who can twist into pretzels or touch their toes with ease. It extends a warm invitation to everyone, regardless of age, ability, or experience. This introduction serves as your gateway into the world of chair yoga, an innovative approach that breaks barriers and opens up a multitude of possibilities for enhancing wellbeing.

Embarking on this path, we understand that the first step towards transformation is often the hardest. Yet, it is also the most crucial. It's about making a commitment to yourself - a promise to embrace a healthier lifestyle. This book is designed not just to instruct but to inspire and motivate you to integrate chair yoga into your life, thereby tapping into a reservoir of vitality and serenity you might not have known existed within you.

Let's dispel the myth that yoga is only for the flexible or fit. Chair yoga brings the essence of traditional yoga into a format that is accessible to all. Through this adaptation, the benefits of yoga, such as improved flexibility, better posture, and decreased stress levels, become available to anyone who is

1

willing to try. Whether you're in an office setting, at home, or even traveling, chair yoga offers the flexibility to maintain your practice.

The beauty of chair yoga lies in its simplicity and adaptability. It requires no special equipment besides a chair and, perhaps, your commitment. This makes it an ideal practice for those seeking a gentle form of exercise that can be adapted to individual needs and fitness levels. As we proceed, we will explore the core principles that make chair yoga an effective tool for enhancing health and wellbeing.

Understanding the roots and evolution of chair yoga enriches our practice, connecting us to a deeper purpose and sense of tradition. While we won't dive deep into its history here, knowing that chair yoga has developed over time to meet contemporary needs adds value to our engagement with the practice.

Many have misconceptions about what chair yoga involves. Some assume it's too easy to provide any real benefits, while others worry they're not "yogi enough" to participate. We're here to debunk those myths and demonstrate how chair yoga can be a powerful tool for everyone. It's about personal progress and using what works for your body.

Starting any new routine can be daunting, but chair yoga is all about finding what works for you. From choosing the right chair to setting up a practice space that invites tranquility, these initial steps are your foundation. While this book will guide you through creating a routine, remember, the best practice is one that you will stick with.

Chair Yoga Essentials

The heart of chair yoga is, undoubtedly, the poses. We'll explore a diversity of movements designed to strengthen, balance, and flex the body, all from the safety and support of a chair. Whether it's a seated forward bend to stretch your spine or a chair pigeon for opening your hips, each pose has been selected for its ability to be modified to fit any level of ability.

Breathing techniques and meditation are integral elements of yoga that enhance the mind-body connection and promote relaxation. Even in a chair, these practices deepen the impact of your physical movements, turning your exercise into a holistic experience that nurtures both body and mind.

Adapting chair yoga for specific needs makes this practice exceptionally inclusive. Whether you're looking for gentle exercises to support rehabilitation, ways to relieve stress, or a midday energy boost, chair yoga can be tailored to address a wide range of goals and challenges.

Incorporating chair yoga into your daily routine is simpler than you might think. With strategies for creating short, effective sequences and tips for practicing at the office or as a break from screen time, we aim to make chair yoga an easy addition to your lifestyle, proving that every little movement counts towards your wellbeing.

Comparing chair yoga to other forms of exercise reveals its unique strengths and versatility. It's an effective, low-impact option that complements traditional exercise routines or serves as a standalone practice. Understanding these nuances will help you to appreciate chair yoga's place in your overall health regimen.

Enhancing your practice with props and modifications ensures safety and maximizes benefits. We're dedicated to empowering you with the knowledge to adjust poses and utilize tools that support your journey, making your chair yoga experience both enjoyable and effective.

Nutrition and wellness go hand in hand with any yoga practice. By linking mindful eating with yoga principles, we extend the philosophy of harmony and balance from the mat (or chair) into everyday life, encouraging a holistic approach to health that nourishes both body and spirit.

Finally, stories of transformation await to inspire and affirm the impact of chair yoga on real lives. These are not just success stories but reminders that we are all on a journey. Wherever you find yourself today, know that movement towards health and flexibility is always possible. With chair yoga, every day is an opportunity to embrace a healthier you, one gentle pose at a time.

Chapter 1:
Chair Yoga Essentials:
Easy Steps to Health and Flexibility

Embarking on a journey to better health and increased flexibility through chair yoga isn't just about trying a new exercise routine; it's about embracing a lifestyle that fosters wellness from the comfort of your chair. This form of yoga, with its specifically designed poses and practices, is an accessible path for anyone looking to improve their physical condition, mental clarity, and overall well-being. Let's dive into what makes chair yoga not just an essential tool for enhancing your life, but an easy and enjoyable one at that.

Chair yoga, at its core, is the adaptation of traditional yoga poses to be performed while seated or using a chair for support. This small adjustment opens up the world of yoga to those who may find standing poses challenging, whether due to age, disability, injury recovery, or simply seeking a low-impact exercise option. However, don't mistake the chair as a limitation; it's your portal to improved strength, flexibility, and mindfulness.

If you're new to chair yoga, you might be thinking, "Is this really for me?" Rest assured, the beauty of chair yoga lies in its versatility. It's designed to cater to individuals at any fitness level or mobility range. Whether you're sitting at a desk all day, recovering from surgery, or you're in your golden years looking to maintain your zest for life, chair yoga can be tailored to meet your needs and goals.

One of the fundamental aspects of chair yoga that we'll explore is the variety of poses available. From gentle stretches that target key areas of tension, like the neck and shoulders, to more dynamic movements that engage and strengthen the core, each pose is a step towards enhancing your physical health. And the best part? These can be done in short bursts throughout the day, fitting seamlessly into your routine.

Chair yoga isn't just about the physical benefits; it's a holistic approach to well-being. Mental health is profoundly impacted by our physical state, and vice versa. Through mindful breathing and meditation techniques integrated into chair yoga practices, you can cultivate a sense of calm, reduce stress levels, and improve your overall mood. Imagine turning a five-minute work break into a revitalising session of self-care.

Understanding the essentials of chair yoga involves recognising it as a bridge to better health, regardless of your starting point. It's about making wellness accessible and enjoyable. The alignment of breath with movement, the focus on flexibility and strength – these principles guide the practice of chair yoga, ensuring that each session enriches your body and mind.

A common hurdle for many when starting any new exercise regimen is the misconception that significant time investment or intensity is needed to see benefits. Chair yoga dismantles this barrier. Even a few minutes a day can lead to noticeable improvements in flexibility, mobility, and well-being. It encourages you to start where you are, use what you have, and do what you can.

Setting yourself up for success in chair yoga is about embracing patience and consistency. Progress might be slow, but it's also steady. Celebrating the small victories – reaching a bit further, feeling a bit more relaxed, breathing a bit deeper – becomes part of the rewarding journey towards a healthier, more flexible you.

As you delve into the world of chair yoga, remember, it's not a solitary path. It's a community, a shared experience among those seeking to improve their quality of life from the comfort of their chair. It's not uncommon for practitioners to forge connections, sharing tips, experiences, and encouragement along the way.

Preparation is key, and choosing the right chair and setting up your practice space are important steps to ensure safety and comfort during your sessions. Be mindful to select a stable chair and create a surrounding area free from distractions, allowing you to focus on your practice and the connection between body and mind.

As you integrate chair yoga into your daily routine, you'll discover it's more than just a set of exercises; it's a philosophy of living well and fostering a harmonious balance between mind and body. It is a testament to the power of adaptability, showing that health and flexibility are achievable goals, regardless of circumstance.

Through the pages of this chapter, we've laid the foundation for your chair yoga journey, highlighting its accessibility, versatility, and bounty of benefits. As we move forward, you'll gain deeper insights into understanding chair yoga, mastering poses, breathing techniques, and how to tailor the practice to your unique needs and aspirations.

So, take a moment to appreciate where you are right now, at the beginning of something truly transformative. Chair yoga isn't just a series of exercises; it's a step towards a more healthful, flexible, and vibrant life. Let's embrace this journey together, with patience, enthusiasm, and the anticipation of the wonders that lie ahead.

Your path to well-being through chair yoga is illuminated with the promise of improved physical strength, enhanced flexibility, and a serene state of mind. It's a journey worth embarking on, a commitment worth making, and a goal within your reach. Let's take that first step together.

Welcome to the world of chair yoga, where every seat is the best seat in the house to embark on your journey toward health and flexibility. Here's to the steps we'll take together, transforming each seated moment into a building block for a better, healthier you.

Chapter 2:
Understanding Chair Yoga

In this chapter, we delve into the essence of Chair Yoga, a practice that stands at the incredible intersection of accessibility and profound transformation. At its core, Chair Yoga embodies the principle that yoga is truly for everyone, dismantling barriers that may have prevented some from exploring the traditional mat-based practice. By using a chair as a primary prop, it extends an invitation to individuals of all ages, health statuses, and mobility levels, ensuring that the myriad benefits of yoga—ranging from increased flexibility and strength to enhanced mental clarity and stress reduction—are within everyone's reach. This inclusiveness not only champions physical well-being but also fosters a sense of community and belonging among practitioners. As we explore the roots and evolution of Chair Yoga in the following sections, we'll uncover its rich lineage and adaptation over time, providing context that underscores its significance in today's wellness landscape. The journey into Chair Yoga is not just about modifying poses; it's about redefining what true inclusivity in health and wellness looks like. Armed with the knowledge of its benefits, we'll debunk common myths, setting the stage for a practice that is as empowering as it is nurturing. Chair Yoga is more than an exercise; it's a beacon of hope, an assurance that wellness is achievable and sustainable, tailor-made for each unique body and the varied lives we lead.

The Origins and Evolution of Chair Yoga

In the journey to embrace a healthier lifestyle, understanding the history and evolution of chair yoga illuminates its significance and adaptability. This form of yoga, which has recently surged in popularity, has deep roots that can enhance our appreciation and practice.

Chair yoga, at its core, is a modification of traditional yoga poses, making yoga accessible to everyone, regardless of physical condition, age, or mobility. This adaptability is central to the spirit of yoga – a practice that has always evolved with time to meet the needs of its practitioners.

The conception of chair yoga is generally attributed to the innovation within therapeutic yoga practices. Yoga teachers began to realize that the benefits of yoga could be extended to those who might not be able to practice on a traditional mat due to health issues, injuries, or disabilities. Thus, chair yoga was born out of necessity, sculpted as a bridge to bring the profound benefits of yoga to a wider audience.

Historically, yoga has always been an inclusive practice. Ancient texts and scholars emphasized the adaptability and personalization of yoga. The invention of chair yoga in modern times is a reflection of this principle, showcasing yoga's dynamic nature and its ability to evolve.

As chair yoga started to gain recognition, it caught the attention of health professionals and therapists who saw its potential as a tool for rehabilitation. It didn't take long for chair yoga to become a recommended practice for those recovering from surgery, dealing with chronic pain, or managing conditions such as arthritis and multiple sclerosis.

What sets chair yoga apart is not just its inclusivity but its simplicity and convenience. The practice doesn't require a large space or specific environment; a chair in your living room, office, or even outdoors suffices. This simplicity has propelled chair yoga into mainstream wellness programs, including those in workplaces, senior centers, and schools.

The evolution of chair yoga continues as yoga instructors innovate and adapt poses for the chair, ensuring the practice remains fresh, engaging, and beneficial. As it evolves, chair yoga instructors are also becoming more skilled in creating sequences that not only address physical health but also mental and emotional well-being.

Technological advancements have also played a role in the spread of chair yoga. Through online classes and social media, people worldwide can now access chair yoga, learn from experienced instructors, and join a global community of practitioners. This accessibility has significantly contributed to the practice's growth and evolution.

Chair yoga's evolution is also evident in its approach to mindfulness and meditation. Initially, the focus was primarily on the adaptation of physical poses. However, as understanding and appreciation for the benefits of mindfulness have grown, chair yoga classes now often incorporate meditation and breathing techniques tailored to seated practice.

One of the most beautiful aspects of chair yoga's evolution is the community and connection it fosters. It brings people together who might not have previously felt welcome in traditional yoga spaces. From seniors to office workers, people are discovering the shared joy and benefits of chair yoga, creating supportive and inclusive communities.

Future directions for chair yoga promise to deepen its impact and reach. With ongoing research into its health benefits, chair yoga is poised to become an even more integral part of holistic wellness practices. Furthermore, as chair yoga instructors innovate and share their practices, the diversity of available sequences and adaptations will continue to grow.

The origins and evolution of chair yoga remind us that yoga is a living practice, one that adapts to meet us where we are. By honoring its history and embracing its potential, we can make the most of this incredibly versatile and inclusive form of yoga. In doing so, we not only enrich our own lives but contribute to the broader evolution of yoga as a practice inclusive of all bodies and abilities.

As we integrate chair yoga into our lives, we're not just practicing a series of poses. We're participating in a rich, evolving tradition that reflects the adaptability and resilience of the human spirit. Chair yoga, with its simplicity and depth, offers a path to wellness that is accessible, effective, and, most importantly, inclusive.

In conclusion, the journey of chair yoga from its therapeutic origins to its place in modern wellness practices exemplifies the transformative power of adaptability and inclusion. By tracing this evolution, we are reminded of the potential within ourselves to adapt, grow, and thrive, regardless of the challenges we may face. Chair yoga is more than a practice; it's a testament to the enduring human capacity for change and wellness.

Benefits of Chair Yoga for Everyone

Chair Yoga is an inclusive practice that welcomes individuals from all walks of life, irrespective of age, fitness level, or physical limitations. This gentle form of yoga, which uses a chair for support, brings a myriad of benefits that contribute significantly to both physical and mental well-being. Let's delve into the numerous advantages that make Chair Yoga a valuable addition to anyone's lifestyle.

Firstly, Chair Yoga boosts flexibility. For many, the word 'yoga' conjures images of complex poses that seem unattainable. However, Chair Yoga demystifies this notion, providing a safe platform for individuals to stretch and enhance their range of motion. This is particularly beneficial as flexibility tends to decrease with age, leading to stiffness and reduced mobility. Through regular practice, participants can notice significant improvements in how they move and feel in their day-to-day activities.

Secondly, practicing Chair Yoga leads to improved strength. Each pose is designed to activate various muscle groups, including those that are often neglected. By engaging in these exercises regularly, practitioners can build and maintain muscle mass, which is crucial for keeping the body strong and resilient against injuries.

Moreover, Chair Yoga promotes better posture. The sedentary lifestyle that is prevalent today has led to widespread postural issues, contributing to back and neck pain. Chair Yoga poses encourage alignment and strengthen the core, which is fundamental in supporting the spine. Consequently, individuals can experience relief from chronic discomfort and enhance their overall posture.

Beyond the physical, Chair Yoga offers profound mental health benefits. It is a form of mindful movement that encourages participants to focus on their breath and body, enabling them to cultivate a sense of mental clarity and peace. This mindfulness practice has been shown to reduce symptoms of stress, anxiety, and depression, making it a powerful tool for emotional well-being.

Chair Yoga also enhances balance, which is essential in preventing falls—a common concern among older adults. Through targeted exercises, individuals can improve their stability and gain confidence in their physical abilities. This aspect of Chair Yoga not only contributes to physical safety but also fosters independence.

Another noteworthy benefit is the accessibility of Chair Yoga. It breaks down barriers to exercise, allowing those with limited mobility, including seniors and individuals with disabilities, to engage in physical activity. Classes can be adapted to meet various needs, ensuring that everyone can participate and reap the health benefits of yoga.

Chair Yoga has also been linked to improved cardiovascular health. Gentle yet effective, the practice can help lower blood pressure, reduce stress on the heart, and improve circulation. These factors are integral to preventing heart disease and promoting overall heart health.

The practice serves as a tool for pain management as well. Regular engagement in Chair Yoga can lead to decreased pain and inflammation, benefiting those with chronic conditions such as arthritis. The gentle stretching and strengthening exercises can make a tangible difference in managing pain levels and enhancing quality of life.

For those concerned about cognitive health, Chair Yoga offers an unexpected boon. The combination of physical exercise and mental focus required during practice can bolster cognitive function, helping to keep the mind sharp and potentially staving off cognitive decline in older adults.

Moreover, Chair Yoga fosters connection. Whether practiced in a group setting or virtually, it provides an opportunity to be part of a community. This sense of belonging can be incredibly uplifting, contributing to a person's emotional and social well-being.

It's also worth noting that Chair Yoga is adaptable. It can serve as a gentle introduction for beginners to the world of yoga or offer an alternative for experienced yogis seeking a less intense practice. Its versatility ensures that it remains relevant and beneficial regardless of one's yoga journey.

Another benefit is its role in enhancing sleep quality. The relaxing nature of Chair Yoga, combined with its physical exertions, promotes better sleep patterns. Participants often report falling asleep faster and enjoying a deeper, more restorative night's sleep after incorporating Chair Yoga into their routines.

Finally, Chair Yoga offers a holistic approach to wellness. It doesn't only address physical health but also touches on nutritional awareness, emotional balance, and spiritual growth. Engaging in this practice encourages a more mindful approach to life, where the harmony between mind, body, and spirit is nurtured.

In conclusion, Chair Yoga presents a myriad of benefits that can enhance one's quality of life on multiple levels. It's more than just a physical practice; it's a journey towards achieving a healthier, more balanced lifestyle. With its adaptability and accessibility, Chair Yoga truly is a practice for everyone, promising a pathway to wellness that is both effective and inclusive.

Debunking Myths About Chair Yoga

As we delve deeper into the world of chair yoga, it's essential to clear the air of some common misconceptions that might be holding potential practitioners back. Many may think chair yoga is too simplistic, not strenuous enough, or only intended for a certain age group. However, these myths couldn't be further from the truth. Chair yoga is a versatile and inclusive practice that can benefit everyone, regardless of age, fitness level, or mobility.

Firstly, let's tackle the notion that chair yoga isn't "real" yoga. Yoga is an ancient practice that focuses on connecting the body, mind, and spirit. This connection can be achieved through various means, including meditation, breathing exercises, and physical postures. Chair yoga incorporates all these elements, simply utilizing a chair as a tool to make yoga more accessible. It's not a watered-down version of yoga; it's a adaptation that makes the discipline inclusive for all.

Another common myth is that chair yoga is only for the elderly or those with limited mobility. While it's true that chair yoga offers excellent benefits for individuals in these groups, its advantages extend to a wide audience. Office workers, frequent travelers, or anyone who finds themselves sitting for long periods can use chair yoga to alleviate the negative effects of prolonged sitting. It's also an excellent way for beginners to start their yoga journey, offering a less intimidating entry point.

Many believe chair yoga doesn't provide a proper workout. This belief underestimates the practice's ability to increase flexibility, strength, and balance. Chair yoga can be as gentle or as challenging as you make it; with the right poses and sequences, you can indeed work up a sweat. The practice also offers unique benefits, such as improving joint health and reducing stress, contributing to overall well-being.

There's a myth that chair yoga is boring. On the contrary, chair yoga can be incredibly dynamic and engaging. With creativity, a chair yoga session can include a variety of poses and sequences that keep the practice interesting and lively. Incorporating props, such as blocks or straps, can add another layer of challenge and excitement to the practice.

Some may think chair yoga doesn't offer the spiritual benefits that traditional yoga does. However, chair yoga can be deeply spiritual. The practice encourages mindfulness, inner peace, and a connection to one's body. It allows practitioners to focus on their breath and be present in the moment, which are key components of achieving a meditative state.

Another myth is that chair yoga can't improve your balance. In fact, chair yoga is an excellent way to safely work on balance. By using the chair as a support, practitioners can confidently explore balance poses they might otherwise find too challenging. This gradual approach helps build stability and confidence over time.

Some think that because you're seated, you can't get a full-body workout with chair yoga. This is not true. Chair yoga poses can target all major muscle groups, from the neck and shoulders down to the legs and feet. By engaging these muscles through various poses and sequences, chair yoga offers a comprehensive workout that touches upon every part of the body.

There's also a misconception that chair yoga is less beneficial than traditional yoga. While chair yoga and traditional yoga have their differences, they share many of the same benefits, such as increased flexibility, improved muscle tone, better stress management, and enhanced mental clarity.

The choice between chair yoga and traditional yoga should depend on personal preferences, goals, and needs.

Lastly, many believe that you need special equipment to practice chair yoga. In reality, all you need is a chair without arms, and you're set to embark on your chair yoga journey. While props can enhance your practice, they're not necessary. Chair yoga's simplicity and accessibility are what make it such a powerful tool for wellness.

By debunking these myths, we open up a world of possibilities for people from all walks of life to experience the transformative power of yoga. Chair yoga is not just a stepping stone to more "advanced" practices; it is a legitimate and complete practice in its own right, offering physical, mental, and spiritual benefits. Whether you're recovering from an injury, dealing with chronic pain, looking to reduce stress, or simply seeking a more accessible way to stay active, chair yoga can be tailored to meet your needs.

Embrace chair yoga with an open mind and let go of any preconceived notions about what yoga should be. With consistency and practice, chair yoga can help you achieve greater health, flexibility, and peace of mind. It's a journey toward wellness that's within reach from the comfort of your chair.

Remember, the essence of yoga lies in the connection with oneself, not in the complexity of the poses. Chair yoga encapsulates this essence beautifully, proving that yoga truly is for everyone. So, push aside those myths and misconceptions and give chair yoga a try. It might just be the thing you didn't know your mind and body needed.

Chapter 3:
Getting Started With Chair Yoga

Embarking on your chair yoga journey is akin to opening a new chapter of wellness in your life. It's not just about the physical poses but also about setting the stage for a transformative experience that nurtures your body, mind, and spirit. Before diving into the vast ocean of chair yoga, the first step is selecting the right chair, a true companion in your yoga practice. It should be sturdy, without wheels, and allowing your feet to rest flat on the floor. Next, you'll want to carve out a serene practice space, one that breathes tranquility into your sessions, free from distractions and conducive to focus and relaxation. Here comes the exciting part – creating a routine that resonates with your personal goals, schedule, and physical needs. This isn't about performing complex poses on day one but about gradually weaving yoga into the fabric of your daily life.

Remember, chair yoga is more than a series of physical poses; it's a gateway to enhanced flexibility, strength, and mental clarity. Starting your practice isn't about perfection; it's about progression. With each session, you'll discover more about what works for you, unlocking the profound benefits of yoga in a way that's accessible, enjoyable, and deeply rewarding. So, let's embrace this journey with an open heart and mind, allowing chair yoga to be your guide towards a healthier, more vibrant you.

Choosing the Right Chair

Embarking on a journey toward health and flexibility starts with some basic but crucial choices, one of which is selecting the perfect chair for your chair yoga practice. Imagine it as choosing a partner in dance – the right match can enhance your performance, while the wrong one could hinder your progress.

First and foremost, your chair should provide a stable, solid seat that can support your movements without wobbling. Stability is key to preventing injuries and ensuring that you can perform each pose confidently. It's not just about safety; it's about creating a foundation upon which your practice can flourish.

The ideal chair has a flat seat. What does this mean for you? It means avoiding those chairs that have a curve or are overly cushioned. These types might be comfortable for sitting, but when it comes to chair yoga, they can alter your alignment and impact the effectiveness of the poses. Supporting your posture starts from the bottom up.

Another essential feature to look for is the absence of arms on the chair. While armrests are great for relaxation, they can get in the way during your yoga practice, limiting your range of motion and the variety of poses you can do. Freeing up space around you encourages freedom of movement and flexibility.

Height is another critical consideration. Your feet should comfortably touch the ground when seated, allowing your knees to form a 90-degree angle. This position promotes good posture and aids in maintaining balance, especially important when engaging in poses that require focus and stability.

Consider the material of your chair. A chair with a bit of texture on the seat can prevent slipping, especially as you move into different positions. However, be wary of materials that are too rough, as they might snag your clothes or even your skin.

Why is weight capacity important? Recognizing the weight capacity of your chair ensures that it can support you securely during your practice. This isn't about body shaming but about fostering a practice environment where you can feel safe and supported in your journey toward health.

The aesthetics of your chair, while not as critical as the other factors, can also play a small role in your practice. Choose a chair that you find visually pleasing if possible. The more you appreciate your practice environment, the more likely you are to stick with your routine. Aesthetics can uplift your mood and motivate you to engage in your practice more frequently.

Before you begin, always check your chair for any signs of wear and tear. Consistently inspecting your chair can prevent accidents and injuries, ensuring that your practice is as safe as it is effective. Your wellness journey should enhance your health, not pose unnecessary risks.

Now, you might wonder where to find such a chair. Look no further than your home or a local store. The beauty of chair yoga is its accessibility. You don't need a fancy yoga chair to get started; many household chairs meet these requirements. The key is to choose mindfully, with an eye toward safety and functionality.

If you're practicing chair yoga in a communal space or a class setting, it's a good idea to arrive a bit early to select the chair that best suits your needs. Taking those extra few minutes to choose can make a significant difference in your experience and the benefits you reap from your practice.

Lastly, remember that the perfect chair is the one that meets your unique needs at this point in your journey. What works for someone else might not work for you, and that's okay. Your practice is your own, and tailoring it to fit your requirements is an essential step toward achieving the health and flexibility goals you've set for yourself.

Inspiring health and flexibility through chair yoga begins with grounding yourself in the right foundation. Choosing the proper chair is not just a preliminary step; it's a vital decision that supports your entire practice. Let your chair be a tool that empowers you to explore the benefits of yoga safely and comfortably. With the right chair and a commitment to your practice, you're well on your way to experiencing the transformative power of chair yoga.

Remember, this journey toward a healthier lifestyle is unique to you, and each choice you make, including the selection of your chair, sets the tone for your practice. Approach this choice with consideration and care, and let it be the first step in a rewarding path toward wellbeing. The right chair awaits you, ready to support you as you embrace the countless benefits of chair yoga.

Setting Up Your Practice Space

Embarking on your chair yoga journey, the ambiance and setup of your practice space can make a vast difference in your experience. Think of your practice space as a sanctuary where stress dissipates, and tranquility reigns. This doesn't mean you need to dedicate an entire room to yoga; a small, dedicated corner will do just fine. The key is to create a space that invites calmness and is free from distractions.

First and foremost, find a spot that feels comfortable. This might be a quiet corner of your living room, a dedicated area in your bedroom, or even a space on your back porch. The importance of natural light cannot be overstated; it uplifts the spirit and enhances your practice. If possible, position your practice space near a window.

Space should be clean and clutter-free. A minimalist environment can help declutter the mind and focus on the present moment. You don't need much – just enough room to extend your arms and legs freely. A tidy space reflects a tidy mind, setting the stage for a more focused and effective practice.

The chair you choose is a cornerstone of your practice. Opt for a sturdy chair without arms, allowing for a range of motion without restriction. Your feet should comfortably touch the ground when seated, ensuring proper alignment. If the chair feels too hard, feel free to add a cushion for added comfort.

Consider the flooring beneath you. While chair yoga can be practiced on any surface, a yoga mat or rug can provide a better grip and delineate your sacred space. It's not just functional; it's symbolic of your commitment to pause and engage in self-care.

Lighting plays a crucial role in creating the right ambiance. While natural light is preferred, soft, artificial light can also create a warm, inviting atmosphere. Avoid harsh fluorescent lights that can strain the eyes and detract from the soothing nature of your practice.

Personalizing your space can significantly enhance your practice. This might include adding a plant for a touch of nature, a small statue or image that inspires peace, or even a scented candle or diffuser with essential oils to engage your senses fully.

Sound can profoundly influence your ability to relax and focus. Consider a small speaker or device to play soothing background music or nature sounds. Alternatively, the sound of a water fountain can add an element of tranquility to your space.

Temperature control is another factor to consider. The room shouldn't be too hot or too cold, as physical comfort is essential to maintaining focus and relaxation. An adjustable fan or space heater can help regulate the temperature to your liking.

Privacy is important. Inform others in your household of your practice time to minimize interruptions. Hanging a "Do Not Disturb" sign or using room dividers can also help create a sense of seclusion and peace.

Accessibility is key. Keep your yoga props, such as blocks, straps, or an extra cushion, within reach. This practical setup ensures a smooth transition between poses and keeps your focus on the practice.

Inspiration can come from surrounding yourself with positive affirmations or motivational quotes placed in your line of sight. These small reminders can serve as powerful tools to uplift your spirit throughout your practice.

Though the aesthetics of your space are important, remember the essence of chair yoga lies in the practice itself. Don't let the quest for a perfect space deter you from starting. The most crucial step is showing up for yourself, regardless of the setup.

Respect the journey and allow your practice space to evolve with you. Over time, you will discover what works best for you, adjusting and adding elements that enhance your experience. Your practice space, like your yoga journey, is unique and personal.

Embarking on your chair yoga journey with a thoughtfully prepared space sets the foundation for a transformative experience. Let this space be your retreat, where you can explore, grow, and find peace within. Your dedication to creating a nurturing environment is a reflection of your dedication to your well-being. Embrace the process, and let your practice flourish in this sacred space you've created.

Creating a Routine That Works for You

Embarking on your chair yoga journey is a thrilling step towards nurturing your body and mind. Let's dive into crafting a personalized routine that resonates with your daily rhythm. Remember, the magic of chair yoga lies in its flexibility and accessibility, making it a perfect match for your unique lifestyle.

The first key to success is setting achievable goals. Ask yourself, what you're looking to gain from your chair yoga practice. Whether it's enhancing flexibility, building strength, or fostering a serene mind, having a clear vision will guide your path forward.

Finding the right time of day for your practice is essential. Are you a morning person, ready to greet the day with energy and enthusiasm? Or, do you find your stride in the evening, unwinding from the day's labors? Listen to your body's natural rhythm and slot your chair yoga practice into a time when you feel most vibrant and receptive.

Creating a comfortable space is equally important. Even a small, designated area can transform into a sacred nook for your practice. Ensure your chosen chair is there, along with any props you might need. This dedicated space will invite consistency and respect for your practice.

Start small. Rome wasn't built in a day, and your chair yoga routine will similarly flourish over time. Initiating your practice with just a few minutes a day can set a foundation, slowly building as you become more comfortable and confident in your abilities.

Variety keeps the practice exciting and covers all aspects of fitness—flexibility, strength, and balance. While it's great to have favorite poses, exploring new ones prevents plateaus and keeps your mind engaged. Remember, every pose has its value and place in your routine.

Listen to your body's feedback. Chair yoga is about nurturing, not straining. If a pose feels uncomfortable, ease off and consider variations or props. This practice is your own, and honoring your body's limits is crucial to a sustainable routine.

Integrate breath work into your routine. The breath is a powerful tool for both calming the mind and energizing the body. Beginning or ending your practice with a few minutes of focused breathing can profoundly affect your overall experience.

Consistency is more critical than duration. It's better to practice for a short time each day than to have an extended session sporadically. This regular engagement helps build a habit, making your chair yoga practice a natural part of your daily life.

Track your progress. Keeping a simple journal or notes on your practice can be incredibly motivating. Over time, you'll be able to see how far you've come, which poses have become easier, and how your goals may have shifted.

Be patient and kind to yourself. Progress in yoga, as in life, is not linear. There will be days when your body seems more cooperative and others when certain poses feel out of reach. This is normal. Recognize and celebrate your efforts rather than focusing solely on outcomes.

Incorporate meditation or mindfulness practices. Chair yoga doesn't end with the physical poses. The inclusion of meditation or mindfulness can round out your routine, offering a comprehensive approach to wellness that nurtures the mind as well as the body.

Seek community and support. Sharing your experiences with others on the chair yoga path can provide encouragement and insights. Whether it's joining a class, participating in online forums, or practicing with a friend, community can be a powerful motivator.

Finally, allow your practice to evolve. As you grow and change, so too will your chair yoga routine. What works for you now might need adjustment down the line. Stay open and flexible to adopting new poses, goals, and practices as you continue on your wellness journey.

In closing, remember that creating a chair yoga routine that works for you is a personal and evolving process. Your practice is a unique expression of your needs, goals, and lifestyle. By listening to your body, setting realistic expectations, and being consistent, you're setting the stage for a rewarding and transformative journey. Chair yoga is more than just a set of poses; it's a pathway to greater health, flexibility, and peace of mind. Embrace it with an open heart and enjoy every step of the way.

Chapter 4:
Essential Chair Yoga Poses

Continuing from mastering the basics and setting up our practice space, we now dive into the heart of chair yoga—its essential poses. Chair yoga, a dynamic version of traditional yoga, adapts poses so they can be done while seated or with the support of a chair. This ensures everyone, regardless of flexibility or mobility, can enjoy the profound benefits yoga has to offer. In this chapter, we'll explore key poses that form the foundation of chair yoga. We start with warm-up poses to gently prepare the body, followed by core strengthening exercises that are not just about building a resilient midsection but also about stabilizing and grounding your entire being. Next, we'll venture into flexibility and balance poses like the Seated Forward Bend and Chair Pigeon, designed to enhance your range of motion and improve your body's equilibrium. Each pose is a step towards unlocking the body's potential, with the chair as a steadfast partner, providing support and stability. Finishing with cooling down poses, we close the practice by allowing the body to relax and absorb the benefits of the session. This chapter isn't just a list of poses; it's a journey toward personal growth and better health. Embrace these poses with an open heart, and let them guide you to a healthier, more balanced lifestyle. These poses lay the groundwork for a practice that not only rejuvenates the body but also calms the mind, proving that the journey to wellness is within everyone's reach, one chair yoga pose at a time.

Warm-Up Poses

Embarking on your chair yoga journey, it's vital to start with warm-up poses that prepare the body for a session of stretches and asanas. These initial movements are designed to gently awaken your muscles, increase circulation, and foster a deeper connection between mind and body. Let's explore how warm-up poses can set a positive tone for the rest of your practice.

Firstly, understand that warm-up poses are not just a prelude but an essential part of the practice. They serve as an invitation for your body to ease into the yoga session. The goal here is not to push but to gently nudge the body, encouraging flexibility and movement without strain. It's important to listen to your body's needs and adapt accordingly.

One of the foundational warm-up poses is the seated mountain pose. Sitting upright, anchor your sit bones in your chair, reach your crown upwards to elongate your spine, and rest your hands on your laps. This pose helps to align your posture and creates awareness of your breath, setting a calm and centered stage for your practice.

Following the seated mountain, introduce gentle head and neck rotations. This not only relieves any tension built up in these areas but also enhances mental clarity. Rotate your head slowly from side to side, and then proceed with gentle neck rolls. Remember, the aim is to treat your body with kindness and respect, avoiding any harsh movements.

Shoulder rolls are next in line. Lift your shoulders up towards the ears and roll them back, encouraging the release of any stiffness within the shoulder region. This movement not only warms up the shoulders but also opens up the chest, promoting better breathing.

Arm stretches further invite warmth and flexibility. Extend one arm across your body, using the other to gently press it towards you, stretching the shoulder. Then, raise your arm overhead, bending at the elbow, and use your opposite hand to press gently, stretching the triceps. Such stretches are crucial in maintaining upper body mobility.

Wrist and finger stretches are often overlooked but are incredibly beneficial, especially in today's keyboard-driven world. Extend your arms forward and gently draw your fingers back towards you, and then, press them downwards. Rotate your wrists in gentle circles, ensuring both directions are covered. Nurturing these small joints can significantly impact your overall comfort and flexibility.

Moving downwards, spinal twists gently engage the core and awaken the spine. Holding onto the back of the chair for support, gently twist your torso to one side, then the other. Ensure this movement originates from the base of the spine, spiraling up, to maximize the stretch and promote spinal health.

Hip and lower back stretches are also integral. A simple way to incorporate this is by gently marching in place, lifting one knee towards the chest at a time. This movement not only mobilizes the hips but also gently engages the lower back, areas often neglected in daily life.

Ankles and toes should not be forgotten. Circle your feet at the ankles, then flex and point your toes. Such movements increase circulation to the extremities and can prevent cramps and discomfort, especially for those who may lead a more sedentary lifestyle.

As you progress through these warm-up poses, maintain a focus on your breath. Deep, intentional breathing not only prepares the body but also the mind, helping to establish a meditative state that can enhance the effectiveness of your practice. Let each inhale invigorate you and each exhale release tension.

Finally, remember that warm-up poses are not just a routine but a bridge to mindful practice. They allow you to transition from the hustle and bustle of daily life into a state of quiet focus and intention. By dedicating time to warm up, you honor the commitment to your health and well-being.

With these warm-up exercises, you're now ready to move into the core of your chair yoga practice. Whether it's strengthening, flexibility, or balance poses, your body and mind are now attuned and prepared for the journey ahead. Let these warm-up poses be a grounding reminder that every journey starts with a single step, or in this case, a gentle stretch.

Embrace the warmth and openness cultivated through these poses as you navigate through your practice. It's this foundation of gentleness and attentiveness to your body's needs that will not only enhance your chair yoga experience but also contribute to a more mindful and health-oriented lifestyle. Welcome to the transformative path of chair yoga, where every pose is an opportunity to explore, learn, and grow.

Core Strengthening Poses

Embarking on a journey toward enhancing your physical health might seem daunting, but with chair yoga, you're taking one of the most accessible and impactful routes. When you focus on strengthening your core, you're building a foundation that supports every other aspect of your movement and well-being. Let's dive into how chair yoga can not only strengthen your core but also transform your overall health.

Core strength is pivotal for more than just physical fitness; it's the epicenter of your body's stability. Whether you're reaching for a high shelf or simply maintaining good posture, a strong core is key. Chair yoga offers a variety of poses designed specifically for core strengthening, all of which can be done from the comfort of a chair.

One fundamental pose is the seated mountain pose, which involves sitting up straight with your feet flat on the floor and engaging the muscles of your abdomen. This pose may seem simple, but it's a powerful way to initiate core engagement and improve posture.

To add a twist, literally, the seated twist pose involves turning your torso to one side while keeping your hips facing forward. This not only strengthens the core but also aids in digestion and detoxification, showing that chair yoga can have holistic health benefits.

Another amazing pose for core strengthening is the seated leg lift. By lifting one leg at a time, just a few inches off the ground, you're engaging the lower abdominal muscles. This pose is deceptively challenging and a testament to the fact that small movements can have a big impact.

For those looking to challenge themselves further, the chair plank pose involves placing your hands on either side of the chair seat and extending your legs behind you, mirroring a traditional plank but with the support of the chair. This variation is intense but incredibly effective for building core strength and stability.

Remember, progress in core strengthening, as in any aspect of fitness, is incremental. Celebrate the small victories, like being able to hold a pose for a few seconds longer or feeling less strain over time. Your body's gradual adaptation to these exercises is a testament to your resilience and effort.

It's crucial to listen to your body throughout your practice. Core strengthening poses should challenge you, but never cause pain. Adjusting your posture or taking a break is not only okay, it's encouraged. Chair yoga is about tuning in to your body's needs and respecting its limits.

Integration of core strengthening poses into your daily routine can have profoundly positive effects on your physical health. A robust core reduces the risk of falls, eases back pain, and improves balance and mobility. The beauty of chair yoga is that these benefits are accessible to everyone, regardless of fitness level.

In addition to physical benefits, focusing on core strengthening can improve mental health. The concentration required for these poses can also serve as a form of mindfulness, helping to clear the mind and reduce stress. This connection between body and mind is a core principle of yoga and a key factor in overall well-being.

Inspiration can be found in every pose, every breath, and every moment of stillness. As you engage in these core strengthening exercises, you're not just building muscle; you're building a foundation for a healthier, more vibrant life. Let each pose remind you of your strength, resilience, and potential for growth.

For those who may be struggling with motivation, remember that every journey begins with a single step—or in this case, a single pose. Imagine the version of yourself that has already achieved your health goals. That version of you exists in the future, and it's your current actions that will bring that future into reality. Let this vision propel you forward.

Engaging with a community, whether in-person or online, can also provide a boost of motivation. Sharing your progress, challenges, and tips with others who are on the same journey can make the experience more enriching and less isolating.

At the heart of core strengthening in chair yoga is the principle of balance—not just physical balance, but balance in our lives. As you work to strengthen your core, you're also learning to balance effort with ease, challenge with self-care, and activity with rest. This holistic approach to health is what makes chair yoga so transformative.

As you continue to explore core strengthening poses in chair yoga, let each session be a stepping stone towards greater health and happiness. The strength you're building goes beyond the physical; it's a testament to your commitment to well-being and a healthier lifestyle. Embrace the journey, and let your strengthened core be a source of stability and power in all aspects of your life.

Flexibility and Balance Poses

In the realm of chair yoga, the Flexibility and Balance Poses chapter serves as a cornerstone for those aiming to enhance their physical and mental equilibrium. These poses, including the Seated Forward Bend and Chair Pigeon, are designed not only to stretch your muscles but also to instill a sense of inner peace and stability in your daily life. Imagine the ease of bending down to tie your shoes or the confidence in navigating slippery sidewalks, all thanks to a few minutes spent on your chair practicing these transformative poses. The beauty of chair yoga lies in its accessibility; you don't need to be a gymnast or a yogi to find your balance and extend your flexibility. Each movement is a step towards breaking the chains of physical constraints, allowing you to move freely and with greater joy. As you incorporate these poses into your routine, you'll discover the remarkable blend of strength and serenity they bring to your body, proving that balance is not just a physical attribute but a harmonious state of being. Embrace each pose with an open heart and mind, and watch as the world around you shifts into a place of greater ease and possibility.

Seated Forward Bend

Transitioning from our discussion on core strengthening poses, let's delve into the Seated Forward Bend, a powerful flexibility and balance pose that's fundamental in chair yoga. This pose, while seemingly simple, carries a wealth of benefits, including stretching the spine and hamstrings, improving digestion, and helping to relieve stress. It's a pose that beautifully illustrates how chair yoga makes traditional yoga poses accessible to everyone.

First, let's discuss the setup. You'll want to start by sitting at the edge of your chair, ensuring your feet can comfortably touch the ground. Keep your spine long and your shoulders relaxed. Your hands should rest gently on your thighs. This initial posture sets the foundation for a successful Seated Forward Bend, promoting both safety and effectiveness.

To execute the Seated Forward Bend, inhale deeply, elongating your spine as if a string were pulling you up from the crown of your head. As you exhale, hinge at your hips and begin to fold forward, leading with your chest. It's crucial to maintain a straight back rather than rounding your spine as you bend. This technique ensures you're stretching properly, protecting your back and maximizing the stretch in your hamstrings.

Go only as far as feels comfortable. For some, this might mean hands resting on the shins; for others, it might involve reaching the ground. The goal is not to force your body into what you perceive the pose should look like but to find a depth of bend that feels good for your body today. Yoga is a personal journey, and chair yoga emphasizes adapting the practice to meet your needs.

Once you find your edge, hold the pose for a few breaths. With each exhale, see if you can deepen the bend, not by pushing but by letting the natural weight of your upper body facilitate the stretch. It's in this holding and breathing where the magic happens—where flexibility is nurtured and the mind begins to quiet.

When you're ready to come up, do so with the same careful attention to form. Inhale and lengthen your spine, using the strength of your core to return to a seated position. You might find it beneficial to place your hands on your thighs for added support as you rise. This mindful return is part of the stretch, allowing your body to absorb the full benefits of the pose.

The beauty of the Seated Forward Bend, and indeed all chair yoga poses, lies in their adaptability. If you find the traditional seated version challenging, adding a prop like a pillow on your lap to "bring the floor to you" can be incredibly helpful. This modification allows you to respect your current flexibility limits while still engaging in the stretch.

Committing to a practice that includes poses like the Seated Forward Bend can significantly impact your flexibility and overall well-being. It's a testament to the power of starting

Mike Ezekiel

where you are and using simple, consistent steps to progress. Each time you practice, you're not just improving your physical flexibility; you're also cultivating a flexible mindset that is open to growth and change.

The psychological benefits of the Seated Forward Bend shouldn't be underestimated. In folding forward, there's a symbolic letting go of stress and worries. It creates a moment of introspection and calm, offering a mental break that can be particularly refreshing during a hectic day. This aspect of the pose exemplifies how chair yoga serves not just the body but the mind as well.

For those dealing with chronic pain or health conditions, the Seated Forward Bend offers a gentle way to stay active. It encourages circulation, aids in digestion, and helps manage stress—all key components of a holistic approach to health. Remember, it's vital to listen to your body and consult with healthcare professionals when incorporating yoga into a health regimen, especially when specific conditions are present.

Incorporating the Seated Forward Bend into your daily routine doesn't require a massive time commitment. Even a few minutes dedicated to this pose can yield benefits. It's a perfect example of how adopting small, healthful habits can lead to significant changes over time. Think of it as planting a seed that will grow with consistent care and attention.

Moreover, the Seated Forward Bend can be an excellent starting point for those new to yoga or anyone looking to deepen their practice. It lays the foundation for understanding how to engage with your body in a mindful, respectful way.

This engagement is at the heart of yoga and a vital step toward achieving greater health and wellness.

Additionally, practicing the Seated Forward Bend can foster a sense of accomplishment. As you notice your flexibility improving and your ability to delve deeper into the pose growing, you'll gain confidence not just in your yoga practice but in your capacity to pursue and achieve wellness goals across your life. This confidence is transformative, influencing how you approach challenges and opportunities daily.

Finally, embracing the Seated Forward Bend within your chair yoga practice is an invitation to explore the broader landscape of yoga. It opens the door to discovering other poses, breathing techniques, and the philosophical aspects of yoga that can enrich your life in myriad ways. Consider it a stepping stone to a deeper, more fulfilling journey toward health and happiness.

As we wrap up our focus on the Seated Forward Bend, remember that the journey to health and flexibility is as much about the mind as it is about the body. Chair yoga, with its adaptability and accessibility, offers a path forward for everyone, regardless of age, fitness level, or mobility. It's a gentle reminder that we all possess the ability to transform our lives, one breath, one pose at a time.

Chair Pigeon

Discovering how to incorporate the Chair Pigeon pose into your routine is more than just a step towards flexibility; it's a leap towards embracing a healthier lifestyle. This pose, traditionally performed on the mat, has been adapted to be accessible from the comfort of a chair, allowing individuals of all abilities to experience its benefits. Today, let's explore this pose, focusing not only on its physical advantages but also on the mental respite it provides.

Chair Pigeon pose, or seated pigeon, targets your lower body, specifically the hips, which are a common area for tension accumulation. In our modern lives, where sitting for prolonged periods is the norm, our hip flexibility can significantly decrease. This pose is a beacon of relief—it unlocks this tension, promoting flexibility and potentially alleviating back discomfort.

Before diving into the specifics, it's essential to select an appropriate chair. This foundational step, crucial for all chair yoga poses, involves choosing a stable chair without wheels, ensuring safety throughout the practice. Remember, the right equipment sets the stage for a successful journey in yoga.

To begin the Chair Pigeon pose, start by sitting upright with your feet planted firmly on the ground, ensuring your spine is aligned. Elegance in posture, from the very start, activates the core and prepares your body for the pose. Breathe deeply, inviting calmness into your practice.

Gently lift your right ankle and place it across your left thigh, just above the knee. This formation creates the shape reminiscent of a pigeon, hence the name. Here, you're already engaging in the act of opening your hips, igniting the path to increased flexibility.

Now, with your hands resting on your shins or the arms of the chair, inhale deeply. As you exhale, lean forward slightly from your hips, enhancing the stretch. It's not about how far you can go but how deeply you can connect with the pose. Honoring your body's limits is a testament to your respect for its capabilities.

Hold this position for several breaths, allowing each exhale to deepen the stretch gently. The beauty of this practice lies in the synergy of breath and movement, a dance that nurtures your body and soothes your mind.

After enjoying the stretch, gently release and return to your original seated position. Take a moment to notice any differences in your body, celebrating the progress made, no matter how small. Replicate the pose on the opposite side, ensuring balance in your practice.

Commitment to regular practice is key; like any worthwhile endeavor, the benefits of the Chair Pigeon pose accumulate over time. Patience and persistence unlock doors to improved flexibility, mobility, and a deeper understanding of your body's language.

Integrating this pose into your daily routine serves as a potent reminder of the importance of self-care. In the hustle and bustle of daily life, setting aside time for Chair Pigeon can be a sanctuary of peace, a haven of tranquility in a chaotic world.

Moreover, this pose's simplicity makes it an ideal entry point for those new to yoga. It demystifies the practice, proving that yoga is truly for everyone, regardless of flexibility or fitness level. Embracing Chair Pigeon is embracing the philosophy that every small step towards health is a victory.

As you continue your chair yoga journey, consider the Chair Pigeon pose not just as an exercise, but as a symbol of transformation. It represents the shift from a sedentary lifestyle to one of active engagement with your well-being. This pose is a testament to the power of adaptability—in yoga and in life.

Remember, the journey to health and flexibility is deeply personal. Comparisons serve no purpose here. Chair Pigeon, with its grace and accessibility, reiterates this principle. It invites you into a space where progress is measured not by the flexibility of your body, but by the openness of your heart and mind.

In conclusion, Chair Pigeon is more than just a pose; it's a pathway to a healthier lifestyle. Through regular practice, not only are the hips liberated from the constraints of modern life, but the mind is also granted the freedom to explore the depths of tranquility. So, embrace this pose with an open heart, and let it guide you towards a life of wellness and joy.

Let this be a reminder that your pursuit of health is a remarkable journey, punctuated by moments of challenge, growth, and profound satisfaction. The Chair Pigeon pose is but one step in this journey, a step that embodies the resilience and adaptability required to thrive. Embrace it with enthusiasm, and let it propel you towards your goals, knowing that each pose, each breath, brings you closer to the life you aspire to live.

Cooling Down Poses

After engaging your body in various strengthening and stretching poses, it's critical to bring your practice to a close with cooling down poses. Cooling down serves the essential purpose of regulating blood flow, gradually lowering heart rate, and bringing your nervous system back to a state of rest. These poses are carefully designed to help you transition smoothly from your practice back into your day with grace and mindfulness.

One of the simplest yet profoundly effective cooling down poses is the **Seated Mountain Pose**. Sit comfortably towards the front of your chair with both feet flat on the ground. Rest your hands on your knees or thighs, and straighten your spine as if a string is pulling you up from the crown of your head. Close your eyes and take deep, slow breaths. Embrace the stability and solidity of the mountain, allowing any residual tension to dissipate with each exhale.

Next, transition to the **Seated Forward Bend**. Inhale deeply, and as you exhale, slowly hinge at your hips, lowering your torso towards your legs. Allow your hands to rest gently on the floor or grasp the legs of the chair for support. This pose aids in calming the brain, reducing stress and anxiety, and stretching the back.

The **Chair Pigeon Pose** is another excellent choice for cooling down. While seated, place your right ankle on your left knee, forming a figure-four shape. Keep your back straight and gently lean forward to intensify the stretch. This pose opens up the hips and lower back, areas that often harbor tension.

Remember to breathe deeply and perform the pose on both sides to maintain balance.

Don't underestimate the power of a good **Twist** to wring out any residual stress. Sit up straight, take a deep breath, and on the exhale, gently twist your torso to the right, using your left hand on the outside of your right knee as leverage. Look over your right shoulder if it's comfortable, and hold for a few breaths before switching sides. Twists are wonderful for stimulating digestion and maintaining spinal health.

Lastly, the **Seated Corpse Pose** is your final stop. Sit comfortably, close your eyes, and let your hands rest on your thighs or in your lap with palms facing up. Take this time to scan your body, noting any sensations without judgment. This pose allows for total relaxation, marking the end of your session and cementing the harmony between mind and body.

As you incorporate these cooling down poses into your chair yoga routine, remember that the goal is not just to stretch muscles but to prepare your mind and body to return to the tasks at hand with renewed energy and a calm demeanor. Cooling down is as much a mental practice as it is physical, inviting mindfulness and a deepened awareness of your body's signals.

Whether you're a seasoned yogi or just starting, respecting this phase of your practice is crucial for overall wellness. It's tempting to rush through or skip cooling down when time is limited, but even a few minutes devoted to these poses can have significant benefits. Investing this time can improve flexibility, decrease muscle soreness, and reduce the risk of injury.

In the broader scope of chair yoga, cooling down is where you reap the rewards of your practice. It's a time for gratitude, reflection, and acknowledgment of your body's work. Let this be a quiet celebration of your strength, flexibility, and persistence.

Remember, consistency is key in chair yoga, as in any form of exercise. The more regularly you can incorporate these cooling down poses into your routine, the deeper their benefits will penetrate, supporting not only physical but emotional and mental well-being.

As you close each session, carry forward the calmness and centeredness you've cultivated. Allow it to infuse the rest of your day with balance and tranquility. The beauty of chair yoga lies in its accessibility and simplicity, proving that profound transformation can come through gentle, patient practice.

Embrace each pose with an open heart and mind, and let your chair yoga journey be a pathway to a healthier, more vibrant life. Cooling down isn't just the conclusion of your practice; it's a bridge to the rest of your day, ensuring you step off the mat (or chair) grounded, refreshed, and ready to face the world with a renewed sense of purpose.

So, as you wrap up your practice, remind yourself of the incredible work you've done. Celebrate your dedication to your well-being. Each pose is a step on the path to a healthier lifestyle, and cooling down is the gentle reminder that in slowing down, we often find our greatest strength and resilience.

Let this segment of your chair yoga practice be an invitation to explore the depths of your inner tranquility. Cooling down is not just a series of poses; it's a practice of self-care, a ritual of calming and preparing oneself for what lies ahead. Let it ground you, let it soothe you, and most importantly, let it empower you to lead a life of balance, health, and wellness.

Chapter 5:
Breathing Techniques and Meditation

As we transition from the physical poses detailed in the previous chapter, let's delve into the cornerstone of any well-rounded yoga practice: breathing techniques and meditation. It's easy to overlook the importance of our breath and the power it holds in calming the mind and rejuvenating the body. Yet, mastering this invisible force can transform your chair yoga experience from merely a physical activity to a profound journey of self-discovery and wellness. Whether you're sitting in your chair feeling tense after a long day or looking for a way to elevate your practice, learning to harness your breath can open doors to a deeper level of physical and mental health. Simple breathing exercises, integrated seamlessly into your chair yoga routine, can significantly enhance your ability to focus, reduce stress, and maintain a serene state of mind. Meanwhile, meditation, though often perceived as daunting by beginners, is nothing more than the art of being present. By incorporating meditation into your practice, you tap into an innate source of peace and clarity that can powerfully impact your overall well-being. This chapter aims to guide you through the initial steps of connecting with your breath and embracing meditation, with the promise that these

51

tools are not only accessible but also instrumental in your journey towards a healthier lifestyle. Through consistent practice, you'll find that these techniques not only enrich your chair yoga experience but also extend their benefits into your daily life, offering a sanctuary of calm in the midst of chaos.

The Role of Breath in Chair Yoga

Embarking on a journey through chair yoga, we often find that breathing isn't just a part of the process; it's the cornerstone of our practice. The act of breathing deeply and intentionally transforms the chair yoga experience, elevating it from a simple sequence of movements to a deeply meditative practice. Let's explore why your breath plays such a pivotal role and how harnessing it can revolutionize your chair yoga sessions.

In the realm of chair yoga, every breath you take is an opportunity to connect more deeply with yourself. It's not merely about filling the lungs with air; it's about breathing life into every part of your body. With each inhale, imagine drawing in fresh energy, and with each exhale, envision releasing tension and fatigue. This visualization not only enhances your physical practice but also clears your mind, creating a sense of calmness and focus.

Consider for a moment the natural rhythm of your breath. It's a rhythm that's as unique to you as your fingerprint. In chair yoga, we tune into this rhythm, allowing it to guide our movements and our pace. This synchronization of breath and movement creates a seamless flow, turning each pose into a gentle dance. The result? A practice that feels more like a moving meditation, leaving you not just physically revitalized, but mentally rejuvenated as well.

Now, let's delve into the therapeutic aspects of breath in chair yoga. Proper breathing techniques can significantly enhance your lung capacity and efficiency, which is a boon for anyone, especially those with respiratory issues or chronic stress. These techniques encourage full oxygen exchange, which can lower blood pressure and induce a state of calm. It's like hitting the body's "reset button," allowing you to tackle stress and anxiety with renewed vigor.

But how exactly do we breathe in chair yoga? It's simple, yet profound. We focus on deep, diaphragmatic breathing—breathing that engages the whole diaphragm and not just the upper chest. This type of breathing is akin to filling a balloon: you start filling it from the bottom, ensuring the foundation is solid before reaching its full capacity. Similarly, diaphragmatic breathing maximizes oxygen intake, energizing and revitalizing the body.

For those new to this concept, fear not. Chair yoga introduces you gently to the art of mindful breathing, making what might initially seem complex, surprisingly accessible. It starts with awareness, with sitting comfortably in your chair and simply observing your natural breath. No judgment, no alteration, just pure observation. This is your baseline, your starting point on the path to mastering the breath.

As you progress, chair yoga teaches you to gently lengthen and deepen your breaths, to control the pace and depth with intention. This control is a powerful tool. It's your anchor during challenging poses, your calm in the midst of life's storms. Learning to command your breath is essentially learning to command your response to any situation, both on and off the mat.

Integration of breath in chair yoga doesn't stop with physical practice. It extends into meditation, serving as a bridge from the physical to the mental. A focused and deliberate breath can draw your attention inward, facilitating a meditative state where thoughts slow down, and clarity emerges. This integration of breathing with meditation is a testament to chair yoga's holistic approach to wellness, addressing both the body and the mind.

This practice of mindful breathing has ripple effects beyond your chair yoga session. It cultivates a sense of presence and mindfulness that enriches every aspect of your life. Imagine facing life's ups and downs with the steadiness and calm that comes from your chair yoga practice. It's a form of resilience that's not just physical but deeply rooted in emotional and mental wellbeing as well.

Moreover, practicing deliberate breath control can empower you in ways you might not expect. It's an affirmation of your ability to influence your own physiology, to calm your mind, and to choose your response to the world around you. This empowerment is a gift, one that chair yoga offers freely, asking only for your willingness to engage in return.

It's remarkable when you think about it—how something as simple and instinctive as breathing can unlock such profound benefits. And yet, in chair yoga, we witness this transformation daily. It's a reminder that sometimes, the most powerful tools are those we carry within us, accessible with just a bit of guidance and practice.

In closing, remember that your breath is your companion in this journey of chair yoga. It's a guide, a healer, and a source of strength. By giving your breath the attention it deserves, you're not just enhancing your chair yoga practice; you're embracing a holistic path toward health and wellness. Let your breath be the foundation upon which you build your practice, your wellbeing, and ultimately, a more vibrant life.

So, as you continue to explore the wonders of chair yoga, let your breath lead the way. Let it inspire your movements, deepen your meditation, and enrich your life. It's a journey well worth taking, and it all starts with a single, mindful breath.

Remember, the power of breath in chair yoga is not just in knowing about it; it's in experiencing it, in living it. It's an invitation to a healthier, more balanced life. Accept it with open arms and an open heart. The journey is yours for the taking, one breath at a time.

Simple Breathing Exercises

Embarking on a journey of health and vitality through chair yoga brings us to a crucial component that intertwines the physical with the mental: breathing exercises. These exercises are not just simple techniques; they are the gateway to harnessing the power of your breath, unlocking a myriad of health benefits that can transform your life.

The essence of breathing exercises lies in their simplicity and accessibility. No matter where you are, your breath is a tool that you can use to calm your mind, reduce stress, and even improve your physical health. It's about turning something we do every minute of every day into a conscious practice that enriches our lives.

Let's start with something called **diaphragmatic breathing**, or belly breathing. This technique encourages full oxygen exchange and can significantly reduce the heart rate and lower blood pressure. Simply sit comfortably in your chair, place one hand on your belly, and breathe deeply through your nose, feeling your diaphragm expand. Then, exhale slowly, observing the fall of your hand. The focus here is on making each breath deeper than the last.

Next is the **4-7-8 technique**, a method that emphasizes not just the breathing itself, but the rhythm of your breath. Breathe in quietly through your nose for 4 seconds, hold your breath for a count of 7 seconds, and then exhale completely through your mouth for 8 seconds. This practice is especially beneficial before bedtime, or during moments of heightened anxiety.

The **alternate nostril breathing**, or Nadi Shodhana, is a yogic breath control practice that harmonizes the left and right hemispheres of the brain, promoting balanced emotional and physical states. With your right thumb, close your right nostril, and inhale slowly through the left. Then, using your right ring finger, close the left nostril, open the right, and exhale. This technique can sharpen focus and relieve stress.

For those moments when you need an instant pick-me-up, try the **energizing breath**, or Kapalabhati. It involves short, powerful exhales and passive inhales. To do this, sit up straight, and with quick contractions of your lower belly, forcefully expel the air from your lungs, allowing them to refill by themselves. This exercise is known to improve alertness and increase energy levels.

But why are these exercises so impactful? The answer lies in their ability to bring you into the present moment, redirecting your focus from the worries and stresses of life to the simplicity and rhythm of your breath. This present-moment awareness is the foundation of mindfulness, a state that has been linked with reduced stress, improved mood, and better focus.

Incorporating these simple breathing exercises into your daily routine doesn't require extra time or special equipment; it just needs your commitment. Even a few minutes each day can make a substantial difference in your wellbeing. Consider it a small investment in your health, with an immense return.

As you practice, remember that patience is key. It's normal for your mind to wander or for certain breathing patterns to feel awkward at first. Gently bring your focus back to your breath without judgment. With time, these techniques will become more comfortable and more impactful.

Challenge yourself to integrate these exercises into different parts of your day. Beyond your chair yoga practice, use them during work breaks, before stressful meetings, or as a soothing end to your day. This constant reinforcement will deepen the benefits, making them more noticeable in your everyday life.

Remember, the goal of these exercises is not perfection but progress. Each day is an opportunity to understand your breath and, by extension, yourself a little better. Embrace each moment, each breath, as a step toward a healthier, more vibrant you.

In the weeks ahead, as you continue to explore and deepen your chair yoga practice, let these breathing exercises be your anchor. Let them remind you that no matter the challenges you face, you have within you the power to calm, to energize, and to transform.

So, take a deep breath, and let's embark on this breath-filled journey together. Through the simple act of breathing consciously, we can unlock the door to a healthier, more mindful existence. Let your breath guide you to depths of wellness you've never imagined possible. The journey is just beginning, and what a beautiful journey it is.

Incorporating Meditation into Your Practice

Embarking on the journey of chair yoga offers a holistic approach to wellness that includes not just physical movements but also practices that nurture the mind and spirit. Among these practices, meditation stands as a cornerstone, empowering individuals to cultivate inner peace, enhance self-awareness, and foster a deep connection with their breath and body. This section delves into how you can seamlessly incorporate meditation into your chair yoga routine, transforming it into a comprehensive practice that nourishes every facet of your being.

Meditation, often misconceived as a daunting task, is, in essence, a simple practice accessible to everyone, irrespective of their experience or background. It's about finding a moment of peace, a quiet in the storm of daily life. Starting small, with just a few minutes a day, can significantly impact your mental and emotional well-being, guiding you toward a more mindful and present state of being.

To integrate meditation into your chair yoga practice, begin by setting a clear intention. Ask yourself, what you wish to achieve through meditation? Whether it's to alleviate stress, enhance concentration, or simply cultivate a moment of peace, this intention will serve as your guiding light, keeping you anchored to your meditation journey.

Choose a comfortable seated position on your chair, ensuring your back is straight and your feet are flat on the ground. This posture aids in keeping you alert and focused during your meditation. Allow your hands to rest gently on your lap, and close your eyes or maintain a soft gaze to minimize external distractions.

Commence your practice by turning your attention inward, observing your natural breathing pattern without attempting to alter it. This focus on the breath acts as the foundation of your meditation, helping you to anchor your mind and find stillness amidst the chaos.

As you sit in meditation, it's natural for your mind to wander, getting caught up in thoughts, plans, or memories.

Whenever you notice this happening, gently guide your focus back to your breath. This practice of returning to the breath fosters patience and kindness toward oneself, enhancing your meditation experience.

Incorporating guided meditations or using a mantra can enrich your practice, offering a structured path to follow. These tools can help in maintaining focus, especially for beginners, making meditation more approachable and less intimidating.

Integrating mindfulness into your practice involves maintaining a moment-to-moment awareness throughout your chair yoga routine. Engage fully with each pose, observing the sensations in your body, the rhythm of your breath, and the thoughts and emotions that arise. This mindfulness practice promotes a meditative state, blurring the lines between movement and meditation.

Conclude your chair yoga session with a few minutes of silent meditation, allowing yourself to absorb the benefits of the practice. This quiet reflection time enables you to connect deeply with yourself, fostering a sense of peace and contentment that you can carry with you off the chair and into your daily life.

Remember, the key to a fruitful meditation practice is consistency. Incorporating meditation into your daily chair yoga routine, even if only for a few minutes, can significantly enhance its benefits, leading to profound transformations in your mental, emotional, and physical health.

In moments of frustration or difficulty in your meditation practice, approach these challenges with compassion and patience. Meditation is a journey, not a destination, and every experience, whether perceived as positive or negative, is an opportunity for growth and learning.

Consider keeping a meditation journal as part of your practice. Recording your experiences, thoughts, and feelings after each session can provide valuable insights into your progress and help you identify patterns or shifts in your well-being over time.

Incorporating meditation into your chair yoga practice isn't just about adding another item to your wellness routine; it's about embracing a holistic approach to health that acknowledges the indissoluble bond between mind, body, and spirit. It's an invitation to slow down, breathe, and connect with the deepest parts of yourself, cultivating a sense of harmony and balance that radiates from within.

As you embark on this journey of integrating meditation into your chair yoga practice, remember that each session is a unique expression of your present state of being. There's no right or wrong way to meditate, only the path that best suits you at this moment. Be kind to yourself, stay open to the experience, and let your practice evolve organically. The benefits you reap, from enhanced mental clarity to emotional stability and increased physical vitality, will serve as a testament to the transformative power of combining chair yoga with meditation.

Let your chair yoga and meditation practice be a sanctuary, a safe space where you can explore the depths of your being, confront your shadows, and emerge more connected, grounded, and at peace. This integrated practice is not just a routine; it's a lifestyle, a philosophy, and a profound tool for personal transformation.

Chapter 6:
Chair Yoga for Specific Needs

Embarking on the journey of chair yoga opens doors to a variety of practices tailored to meet the unique needs and challenges that everyone faces. Whether you're navigating the limitations of mobility, the stresses and strains of daily life, or simply seeking an energizing boost to revitalize your midday slump, chair yoga offers adaptable, accessible solutions. This chapter delves into how chair yoga can be specifically catered to empower individuals, providing the tools to transform daily challenges into opportunities for growth and well-being. From adaptations that make yoga inclusive for all to targeted practices designed for stress relief and energy renewal, we'll explore how to integrate these specialized sequences into your routine, ensuring that your practice not only fits into your life but also enriches it profoundly. Incorporating chair yoga for specific needs isn't just about adapting the practice; it's about embracing a healthier lifestyle that acknowledges and celebrates your unique journey towards wellness.

Adaptations for Limited Mobility

If you're diving into this section, it's possible you're seeking a way to make yoga accessible and rewarding, despite facing challenges with mobility. *This isn't just about making do,* it's about tailoring a practice that empowers and respects your body's needs. Chair yoga isn't merely an alternative version of traditional yoga; it's a full-fledged practice designed to enhance flexibility, strength, and mental clarity for those who find standard poses challenging.

Understanding that limited mobility does not equate to limited capability is the first step in adopting this empowering mindset. **Every body** has potential, and chair yoga helps unlock that. Whether it's due to age, injury, or a chronic condition, acknowledging where you're at today without judgment is crucial. It's about focusing on what you can do and exploring your practice from there.

Let's talk setup. Choosing the right chair is pivotal. It should be stable and comfortable, with your feet flat on the ground when seated. This base is your launching pad into a world of poses and sequences designed to cater to your specific needs. It's your ally in ensuring safety and support as you journey through your practice.

Creating a routine that feels *personal* to you is another key aspect. The beauty of chair yoga lies in its versatility. Maybe today you focus on upper body stretches, and tomorrow, you explore breathing techniques that help center your mind. There's a rich tapestry of exercises at your disposal, each adaptable to suit your energy levels and physical capabilities on any given day.

Breathing, an essential element of all yoga practices, takes on a new dimension in chair yoga. It's not just a bridge between mind and body; it's a tool for deepening your practice and navigating the challenges of limited mobility with grace and perseverance. Simple breathing exercises can significantly enhance your sense of well-being, both during and outside of your practice.

Adaptations to traditional yoga poses can illuminate new paths to flexibility and strength. The Seated Forward Bend, for instance, highlights how slight modifications ensure that everyone can experience the benefits of each pose. It's not about reaching the floor; it's about moving in a way that feels right for you, creating space within the body and mind.

Chair Pigeon offers another example of adaptation that respects and acknowledges limited mobility. This pose opens up the hips and lower back, areas that can suffer from prolonged sitting or limited physical activity. It's a gentle reminder that mobility, no matter its range, can always find room for improvement and care.

Let's not overlook the power of cooling down poses and how they can be adjusted to suit chair yoga practitioners. These movements and stretches signal to your body and mind that it's time to re-ground after your practice, fostering a sense of completion and serenity.

Incorporating meditation into your chair yoga routine enriches the practice even more, acting as a powerful ally in your journey toward mental clarity and emotional balance. The chair offers a unique support for meditation, allowing you to maintain an aligned posture that encourages focus and inner peace.

As you continue to explore and adapt chair yoga to your needs, remember that every movement, no matter how small, is a step toward enhancing your well-being. It's a process of learning and adapting, discovering what works best for you, and recognizing the progress in your journey, not just the destination.

Integrating chair yoga into your daily routine provides a structured, yet flexible approach to maintaining your health and wellness. Short sequences can be powerful tools for managing stress, boosting energy, and maintaining joint health – all from the comfort of your chair.

Cultivating a practice that's both fulfilling and safe means being mindful of your body's signals. Adapting poses, adjusting the length of your practice, and using props are all strategies that prioritize your well-being. Remember, it's okay to take things gradually, building up strength and flexibility at your own pace.

Exploring chair yoga also opens the door to a community of practitioners who share similar paths. Many find encouragement and motivation in the stories of others who have adapted yoga to meet their needs, showcasing the transformative power of this practice.

Last but not least, practicing chair yoga is a testament to the resilience and adaptability inherent within all of us. It embodies the principle that yoga is truly for every body, offering a path to wellness that is both inclusive and accessible. So, as you embark or continue on your chair yoga journey, remember to celebrate each moment on the mat (or chair) as a step toward a healthier, more vibrant you.

Chair Yoga for Stress Relief

In today's fast-paced world, stress has become an inevitable part of our lives. The quest for a serene mind and a stress-free life leads many to explore various avenues, one of which is chair yoga. This section delves into how chair yoga can be a potent tool for alleviating stress, offering a haven of tranquility in the midst of chaos.

Firstly, let's understand what stress really does to our body. When we're stressed, our body goes into a 'fight or flight' mode which, in the long run, can wear us down, affecting our health adversely. Here, chair yoga steps in as a gentle yet effective method to combat stress. Its accessibility ensures that anyone, regardless of their physical condition, can practice and reap its benefits.

Chair yoga, at its core, combines the principles of mindfulness with physical movement. This combination is key to managing stress. Through mindful breathing and gentle stretches, chair yoga helps in calming the mind, bringing a sense of peace and relaxation. It enables us to be present in the moment, driving away anxieties and worries that plague our mind.

The beauty of chair yoga lies in its simplicity. It doesn't require extensive preparations or gear – just a chair and a few minutes of your day. This simplicity makes it an ideal stress-relief tool for those who have hectic schedules and can't find time for longer yoga sessions. Even a few minutes of chair yoga during a break at work can significantly lower stress levels.

Let's embark on this journey together and explore some chair yoga poses specifically designed for stress relief. One fundamental pose is the seated mountain pose, which involves sitting tall and breathing deeply, aligning your body and mind. This pose is a great starting point to encourage deep breathing and foster a state of calmness.

Another vital pose is the seated forward bend. This pose allows you to stretch your back and neck gently, areas where stress tends to accumulate. By bending forward, you create space in your spine, encouraging relaxation and releasing tension.

The beauty of these poses is that they can be integrated seamlessly into your daily routine. Whether it's a quick session in the morning to start your day on the right note or a few minutes during your lunch break to alleviate midday stress, chair yoga offers flexibility and convenience.

Breathing exercises form an integral part of chair yoga and stress management. Simple techniques like deep belly breathing or alternate nostril breathing can be immensely effective in calming the mind and reducing stress. These exercises can easily be done while seated, making them a perfect fit for chair yoga routines.

Incorporating meditation into your chair yoga practice adds another layer of stress relief. Meditation encourages mindfulness and helps in managing stress by teaching us to detach from our worries and thoughts, allowing us to gain a broader perspective on our problems.

The cumulative effect of regular chair yoga practice is profound. Over time, you might notice a significant reduction in your stress levels, a deeper sense of peace, and an improvement in your overall quality of life. Chair yoga teaches us that managing stress is not always about changing the external circumstances but about altering our internal response to those circumstances.

Chair yoga for stress relief is not just about the physical poses; it's also about cultivating a positive mindset. It encourages us to slow down, breathe, and reconnect with ourselves. This mental shift is crucial for long-term stress management and overall well-being.

Remember, the goal is not perfection but progress. Chair yoga is a journey, and every gesture, no matter how small, is a step toward a more peaceful and stress-free life. Be kind and patient with yourself as you explore this path.

Let chair yoga be your sanctuary in the hustle and bustle of daily life. Use it as a tool to combat stress, to find your calm in the chaos. With regular practice, chair yoga can help you navigate life's challenges with greater ease and resilience.

In conclusion, chair yoga for stress relief is much more than a series of poses. It's a holistic approach to well-being that combines physical movement, breathing exercises, and meditation. It's about creating harmony between the body and mind, enabling us to live a more balanced and stress-free life.

Embrace chair yoga into your life and discover the transformative power it holds in managing stress.

As we move forward in our chair yoga journey, let's carry the lessons of simplicity, mindfulness, and self-compassion with us. Let these practices be a source of strength and serenity, guiding us toward a healthier, more centered existence.

Energizing Poses for Midday Boosts

Let's face it, we've all been there - the midday slump. It sneaks up on you, and suddenly, you're five cups of coffee deep, trying to shake off that drowsy feeling that's been dragging you down since lunch. But before you reach for that next cup of java, consider the transformative power of chair yoga to revitalize your afternoon. Chair yoga, with its unique set of poses designed for midday boosts, can be your secret weapon against the afternoon blues.

The beauty of chair yoga is that it's incredibly accessible; whether you're in a bustling office, a quiet home, or even on the go. These energizing poses are specifically designed to invigorate your body and mind, helping you power through the rest of your day with ease and positivity. So let's dive into this wonderful practice and explore some key poses that will leave you feeling refreshed and charged.

First up is the "Seated Mountain Pose," a fundamental pose that establishes the foundation for all other chair yoga poses. It's all about alignment and creating space in your body. Sit up straight, grounding your feet firmly on the floor, and reach your arms upwards, stretching towards the sky. Feel the energy coursing through your body as you breathe deeply, letting this simple yet powerful pose awaken your senses.

Next, we transition into the "Chair Sun Salutation," a mini sequence that mirrors the energizing flow of its traditional counterpart. This sequence involves a series of gentle stretching and bending movements, all performed while seated. It's designed to warm up the body, boost circulation, and shake off any stiffness or lethargy. Embrace the fluidity of your movements and let each breath guide you deeper into the sequence.

Another gem in the roster of energizing poses is the "Seated Twist." This pose not only revitalizes the spine but also stimulates the digestive system, which can often become sluggish during the midday lull. Twist gently from your core, respecting your body's limits, and use your breath to deepen the stretch with each exhale. It's a quick pick-me-up that leaves you feeling rejuvenated.

"Chair Cat-Cow" brings flexibility and fluidity to your spine, mimicking the movement of a waking cat stretching languorously in the morning sun. This pose encourages you to move your spine from a rounded position (Cat) to an arched one (Cow), promoting spinal health and vitality. The rhythmic movement in sync with your breathing acts as a gentle wake-up call for your body.

For an extra boost, try the "Seated Eagle Pose," which is fantastic for releasing tension in the shoulders and neck - common areas where stress accumulates. The act of crossing your arms and legs in this pose helps to enhance focus and concentration, pulling your mind back from its afternoon wanderings to a state of sharp alertness.

Don't forget to incorporate the "Chair Warrior" series to empower and energize your entire being. These poses help build strength, focus, and determination, embodying the warrior spirit within. As you strike these poses, feel the surge of energy replacing any feelings of fatigue or weakness.

The importance of breath cannot be overstated in chair yoga. Integrate "Breath of Joy" – a dynamic breathing exercise that invigorates the body and clarifies the mind. Its rhythmic nature is uplifting, ensuring that you're well-armed to tackle any challenges the day might throw your way.

"Chair Forward Bend" is a wonderful pose to conclude your midday session. It calms the nervous system and helps in reducing stress and anxiety. Allow yourself to fold forward, releasing the tension from your back and shoulders, and let the gentle pressure on your abdomen soothe your digestive system.

Incorporating these poses into your daily routine can significantly transform your afternoon slump into a period of productivity and vigor. It's amazing how a short chair yoga session can recalibrate your energy levels, offering a natural and healthy alternative to caffeine or sugar-laden solutions.

Remember, the key to reaping the benefits of chair yoga lies in consistency and mindfulness. Make a conscious effort to integrate these poses into your daily schedule. Even a few minutes can make a profound difference in how you feel and function.

Chair Yoga Essentials

Chair yoga is not just about the physical poses; it's a holistic approach that encompasses mind, body, and spirit. As you practice, focus on fostering a positive mindset, embracing gratitude for what your body can do, and cultivating an inner sense of peace and contentment.

So, the next time you feel that midday slump creeping up on you, turn to your chair yoga practice. Let it be your bridge over the energy lull, guiding you back to a place of vitality and inspiration. With every pose, remember that you're not just going through the motions; you're nurturing your well-being and enhancing your life, one breath at a time.

In closing, chair yoga for midday boosts is more than just a series of poses; it's a lifestyle choice that champions self-care and wellness. By incorporating these poses into your routine, you're making a powerful statement about valuing your health and vitality. It's a journey of transformation that starts with a simple seat and unfolds into a richer, more vibrant life experience.

So go ahead, give yourself the gift of energizing chair yoga. It's a choice that supports not only your physical health but also your mental clarity and emotional balance. Here's to conquering the afternoon slump and embracing a life filled with energy, joy, and wellness.

Chapter 7:
Integrating Chair Yoga into
Your Daily Routine

Let's dive into how chair yoga can seamlessly blend into the fabric of your day, irrespective of how packed your schedule seems to be. Think of chair yoga not as an addition to your to-do list, but as a natural integration that enhances your daily living. It's about making your health and well-being a priority without overwhelming your routine. Begin by identifying moments throughout your day that are naturally suited for a brief pause—these can be your golden opportunities for a quick chair yoga sequence. Whether it's a few minutes in the morning to ground yourself before the hustle begins, a midday break to relieve the tension that accumulates from hours of desk work, or a calming sequence before bed to ensure a restful sleep, chair yoga can be your go-to tool for maintaining balance. It's about creating short, effective sequences that you can easily remember and look forward to. Moreover, incorporating chair yoga at the office and using it as an intentional break from screen time not only boosts your productivity but also safeguards your posture and well-being. By making chair yoga a natural extension of your daily routine, you embrace a lifestyle that prioritizes health, flexibility, and mental clarity—transforming the ordinary into an ongoing journey toward wellness. Let chair yoga be your ally in navigating the demands of modern life with grace and strength.

Creating Short, Effective Sequences

Incorporating chair yoga into your daily routine doesn't have to be a daunting task. In fact, creating short, effective sequences can seamlessly integrate this form of exercise into your life, offering numerous benefits without requiring a significant time commitment. Let's dive into how these concise practices can be your gateway to a healthier lifestyle.

Firstly, understanding the essence of chair yoga allows for the creation of sequences that are not only brief but impactful. Chair yoga, a gentler form of yoga, makes the practice accessible to everyone, regardless of fitness level or mobility. By utilizing a chair, it provides stability and support, making poses easier to perform while still offering the core benefits of traditional yoga, such as flexibility, strength, and stress reduction.

To begin crafting these sequences, identify the primary goal you wish to achieve through your practice. Whether it's to energize your body in the morning, provide a midday stress relief, or unwind before bed, setting your intention guides the selection of poses that align with your objective. Each sequence can be tailored to meet your specific needs, making your practice highly personalized and effective.

Start with a warm-up to loosen the body and prepare it for the practice ahead. Simple neck rolls, shoulder shrugs, and arm raises can be done right in your chair and don't take more than a few minutes. These movements increase blood flow and prepare your muscles for a deeper practice.

Following the warm-up, choose a core set of poses that address the body areas you're focusing on. For a sequence designed to boost energy, incorporate poses that open the chest and stimulate the spine, like seated twists and chair cat-cow stretches. If relaxation is your aim, opt for poses that promote a sense of calm, such as seated forward bend and chair pigeon pose.

Each pose should be held for a few breaths, emphasizing mindful breathing which enhances the yoga practice's mental benefits. Remember, the quality of the pose is more important than the quantity. Performing a few poses with intention is more beneficial than rushing through a longer sequence.

Incorporating transitions between poses smoothly turns your practice into a fluid sequence that keeps the body engaged and mind focused. Think of your movements as a dance, where each movement flows into the next, keeping your body in a state of graceful motion.

To conclude your sequence, always include a cool-down phase. This could involve a brief meditation or simple breathing exercises. This final step allows your body to assimilate the benefits of your practice, transitioning you into a state of relaxation or, depending on your goal, leaving you energized and ready to tackle the rest of your day.

Timing is key in creating short, effective sequences. Even five to ten minutes a day can yield significant benefits. Use a timer if you're pressed for time, ensuring you stay on track and complete your practice within your allotted window.

Variety not only adds interest but can also enhance the effectiveness of your practice. Rotate through different sequences or modify the poses to target various areas of the body and mind. This approach keeps your practice fresh and engaging, encouraging consistent practice.

For those integrating chair yoga into a busy lifestyle, it's essential to remain flexible with your practice. Some days might allow for a longer session, while others might only spare a few minutes. The beauty of chair yoga lies in its adaptability; even the shortest sequences can contribute to your overall well-being.

Document your practice to monitor your progress and understand the patterns in your sequence preferences. Reflecting on your journey can be incredibly motivating, showcasing how even small, consistent efforts lead to meaningful change.

Finally, remember that the goal of integrating chair yoga into your daily routine is to enhance your quality of life. It's not about perfection or achieving the most advanced poses. Embrace the journey, listen to your body, and appreciate the moments of clarity and calm that your practice brings.

In conclusion, creating short, effective sequences in chair yoga can vastly improve your health, flexibility, and mental well-being. By making these practices a regular part of your day, you invite balance, strength, and serenity into your life.

Embrace this gentle form of yoga and watch as it transforms your daily routine, one pose at a time.

Embarking on this journey requires no extensive preparations—just a chair, a few minutes, and a commitment to your well-being. Start today, and let chair yoga be your guide to a healthier, more balanced lifestyle.

Chair Yoga at the Office

Stepping into the bustling energy of an office, with phones ringing and keyboards clacking, it might seem impossible to carve out a moment for peace and well-being. Yet, here lies the perfect backdrop for integrating chair yoga into your daily routine. Think of chair yoga as your secret weapon against the stress and sedentary nature of office life. It's accessible, discreet, and most importantly, effective in promoting health and flexibility without leaving your desk.

Imagine the transformative power of inserting short yoga sessions into your workday. It's not just about stretching; it's about re-centering, recharging, and reinforcing a connection between mind and body that often gets lost in the shuffle of deadlines and meetings. The beauty of chair yoga is its simplicity and adaptability, making it a seamless addition to your office environment.

The first step is acknowledging the opportunities your office chair offers beyond just a place to sit. It becomes your tool for grounding, balance, and flexibility. With a focus on posture, breathing, and mindful movement, even a few minutes of chair yoga can result in significant benefits, such as increased focus, decreased stress, and improved posture.

To get started, you don't need any special equipment—just your chair and a willingness to take a brief pause from the digital world. Begin by setting a regular reminder to take short yoga breaks. Consistency is key to forming a habit, and even a few minutes can make a difference.

A simple way to integrate chair yoga is to begin with breathing exercises. Deep, deliberate breaths can help clear your mind and reduce stress, setting the stage for physical poses. Follow your breath with a series of gentle neck and shoulder stretches to ease tension that accumulates from sitting at a desk. These movements not only soothe but also prepare the body for more dynamic poses.

Next, incorporating seated twists and side stretches can help reinvigorate your spine and encourage flexibility. These poses can be done discreetly, without drawing attention, making them perfect for the office environment. Each pose can be held for a few breaths, focusing on the stretch and relaxation of the muscles.

Chair pigeon pose, adapted for seated practice, targets the hips and lower back, areas that often suffer from prolonged sitting. This pose can be done at any point during the day to relieve tightness and promote mobility. It's a reminder that mobility work isn't confined to the gym or yoga studio—it's necessary wherever we find ourselves seated.

One of the unique aspects of chair yoga is the opportunity to incorporate mindfulness practices seamlessly. Between poses, take moments for mindful breathing or a short meditation, harnessing the calm within the office chaos. This practice enhances focus and productivity, making the transition back to work smoother and more efficient.

Engaging in chair yoga also promotes a mindful approach to the workday, encouraging breaks that are both physically and mentally restorative. It shifts the perspective on breaks, from time lost to essential moments that contribute to long-term productivity and well-being.

In motivating yourself to practice chair yoga, remember the cumulative effect of regular movement. Every stretch, twist, and breath contributes to a more flexible, vibrant, and healthy body. It's an investment in your health that pays dividends in energy, focus, and resilience.

For those concerned about drawing attention or disrupting the office environment, consider starting a chair yoga group among interested colleagues. This not only normalizes the practice but also fosters a community of well-being within the workplace. Together, you can share sequences, experiences, and motivation, turning what might have been solitary breaks into a shared journey toward health and flexibility.

Implementing chair yoga at the office doesn't require drastic changes to your schedule or physical space. It's about making the most of the opportunities presented by your existing environment. With each pose, breath, and moment of mindfulness, you're not just doing yoga; you're integrating a practice of well-being into every aspect of your day.

As you continue with chair yoga, notice the shifts in your body and mind. The aim is not perfection but progress and presence. Celebrate the small victories, like feeling less stiff after a long day of work or finding yourself more focused and less frazzled amidst the office buzz.

Remember, chair yoga at the office is more than just a series of poses; it's a statement about prioritizing your health and well-being, even in the least likely of places. It demonstrates that balance and flexibility, both physical and mental, can be cultivated and maintained anywhere, even at your desk. Let chair yoga be your gentle, empowering ally in navigating the demands of office life, guiding you to a healthier, happier you.

In conclusion, integrating chair yoga into your office routine is a simple, effective way to combat the challenges of a sedentary lifestyle and work-related stress. It's your toolkit for fostering agility, serenity, and wellness in the unlikeliest of environments. So take the leap, embrace the practice, and transform your desk into a sanctuary of health and well-being. Your body, mind, and spirit will thank you.

Using Chair Yoga as a Break from Screen Time

In today's digitally dominated world, our eyes and minds are relentlessly glued to screens, be it for work, education, or leisure. The constant screen time not only strains our eyes but also our bodies, tethering us to a cycle of sedentary habits. However, integrating chair yoga into your daily routine, especially as a break from screen time, can be a game-changer for your overall well-being.

Chair yoga, a versatile and accessible form of yoga, offers an effective respite. It allows individuals to engage in physical activity without needing to step away from their work environment. This section dives into how you can seamlessly weave chair yoga into your day, particularly to counteract the physical and mental weariness from excessive screen time.

Firstly, acknowledge the need for breaks. Understand that your productivity and focus naturally decrease after prolonged periods of screen time. Scheduling short chair yoga breaks can rejuvenate your senses, improve circulation, and refocus your mind. It's about giving yourself permission to pause and reset.

Commence with gentle neck rolls. Given the forward-facing nature of screen work, our necks bear a considerable amount of stress. Sit up straight in your chair, slowly lower your chin to your chest, and gently roll your head in a circular motion. This simple move can alleviate tension in your neck and shoulders.

Next, engage in a seated twist. Place your right hand on the back of your chair and your left hand on your right knee. Inhale deeply, lengthening your spine, and as you exhale, twist your torso to the right. This twist detoxifies your organs and relaxes your spine — a perfect antidote to hours of sitting.

Incorporate a seated cat-cow stretch. Place your hands on your knees, inhale as you arch your back and look upwards, then exhale as you round your spine, pulling your belly in. This movement not only flexes your spine but also fosters deeper breathing, inviting more oxygen into your body, invigorating your energy levels.

Don't overlook your wrists and fingers, often strained from typing and clicking. Stretch your arms out in front of you, palms facing down, and gently fold your wrists downwards and upwards. Make fists and roll your wrists in circles, then stretch your fingers wide. These simple exercises can prevent carpal tunnel syndrome and reduce stiffness.

Embrace the seated mountain pose for a moment of stillness and grounding. Sit at the edge of your chair, feet flat on the ground, and extend your spine tall. Rest your hands on your thighs and take deep, calming breaths. Close your eyes if comfortable, and let this pose center your mind, pulling it away from digital disturbances.

Leverage the benefits of guided visualization during your chair yoga breaks. With your eyes closed, envision a serene setting — perhaps a quiet beach or a sunlit forest. Such mental escapes can significantly lower stress levels, offering a refreshing mental break from the hustle of digital realms.

Practicing these simple chair yoga sequences can profoundly impact your fight against the adverse effects of prolonged screen time. It not only offers a physical stretch but also a mental break, fostering a refreshed and balanced state of being.

Remember, the key to successful integration of chair yoga as a break from screen time is consistency. Make it a habit to take these pauses, setting reminders if needed. These short durations of disconnection will lead to longer periods of concentrated and productive work or study.

Additionally, encourage others in your workspace or home to join in. Creating a shared experience can enhance the sense of community and accountability, making the practice even more rewarding.

Finally, personalize your chair yoga breaks. Listen to your body and adjust the movements and duration according to your needs. What works best for you is what will make this practice a sustainable and enjoyable part of your daily routine.

In conclusion, leveraging chair yoga as a break from screen time is not just an investment in your physical health but a profound dedication to your mental and emotional well-being. It's a powerful tool in your arsenal to combat digital fatigue, elevate your mood, and enhance your productivity in a holistic manner. Embrace this practice, and you'll find yourself navigating the digital world with greater ease, balance, and vitality.

As you close your laptop or put down your phone to transition into your next chair yoga break, remember that each movement, each breath, is a step towards a healthier, more centered you. Let chair yoga be the bridge between your digital and physical worlds, harmonizing them into a lifestyle that supports your well-being from every angle.

Chapter 8:
The Pros and Cons of Chair Yoga
Compared to Other Exercises

Finding a fitness routine that sticks can often feel like navigating a labyrinth, especially when you're weighing the benefits of chair yoga against the myriad of other exercises available. Chair yoga, a gentle yet effective form of yoga, offers unique advantages, particularly for those seeking low-impact options or needing a practice that's accessible regardless of mobility issues. It stands out by enhancing flexibility, improving muscle strength, and reducing stress, all without requiring participants to get down on a mat. This makes it a peerless choice for individuals who spend much of their day seated or who find traditional yoga poses challenging.

However, chair yoga isn't without its limitations. While it excels in providing a safe and inclusive environment for exercise, those looking for high-intensity workouts that significantly raise the heart rate might find it less fulfilling. In comparison to activities like brisk walking, swimming, or cycling, chair yoga might not deliver the same level of cardiovascular benefits. Yet, it's important to remember that chair yoga offers a holistic approach, focusing on the mind-body connection and breathing techniques that can enhance overall well-being in ways that purely physical exercises might not.

Engaging with chair yoga also offers the unique benefit of adaptability. Its poses and sequences can be modified to suit your personal needs and goals, making it a versatile tool in your wellness arsenal. Whether you're looking to find a gentle introduction to fitness, seeking stress relief, or need exercises that accommodate mobility limitations, chair yoga provides an accommodating pathway. However, defining your personal health and fitness objectives is crucial in determining if chair yoga aligns with your goals or if it should complement other forms of exercise in your regimen.

Ultimately, the choice between chair yoga and other exercises hinges on a blend of personal preference, health considerations, and fitness goals. While it may not replace high-intensity cardiovascular workouts, chair yoga fills a vital niche, emphasizing mental clarity, flexibility, and strength, which supports a well-rounded approach to health. Embrace the journey towards wellness by considering how chair yoga might fit into your life, remembering that the best exercise is not only about the physical benefits but also about finding joy and sustainability in the practice.

Chair Yoga vs. Traditional Yoga

In the quest for a healthier lifestyle, you may find yourself at a crossroads between traditional yoga and chair yoga. Both offer incredible benefits that can guide you toward greater health and flexibility, yet they cater to different needs and abilities. Let's take a deeper dive into how chair yoga stands next to its traditional counterpart, helping you determine which path might best support your journey toward wellness.

Traditional yoga, known for its physical demands, requires participants to engage in poses on a mat, often moving through sequences that can challenge both the body and mind. It has been celebrated for centuries for its ability to improve flexibility, strength, and mental clarity. However, it's not accessible to everyone. For those with mobility issues, injuries, or age-related concerns, the prospect of participating in traditional yoga can feel intimidating, if not wholly unreachable.

This is where chair yoga enters the scene, a gentler form of yoga that makes the practice accessible to a broader demographic. Chair yoga modifies traditional poses to be performed while seated or with the aid of a chair, significantly reducing the strain on muscles and joints. It offers a passage to the benefits of yoga without the necessity of getting down on a mat, making it an inclusive option for people of all ages and fitness levels.

One of the most compelling contrasts between chair yoga and traditional yoga is the accessibility factor. Chair yoga opens the door for individuals who thought yoga was out of their reach. Whether it's due to chronic pain, disability, or simply a fear of not being "flexible enough," chair yoga proves that yoga can truly be for everyone.

Mike Ezekiel

Despite being a gentler form, chair yoga does not compromise on the benefits. Participants can still enjoy improvements in flexibility and muscle tone, enhanced respiratory and cardiovascular health, and a reduction in stress and anxiety. These advantages mirror those found in traditional yoga practices, making chair yoga not just a modified form of yoga but a potent one in its own right.

Nevertheless, aficionados of traditional yoga might argue that certain aspects of the practice cannot be fully replicated in a chair-based setting. The intrinsic connection between the body and the earth, experienced in many mat-based poses, is seen as a foundation for grounding and centering oneself in traditional yoga. While chair yoga offers superb adaptations, this particular element may differ in its intensity and approach.

When considering the social aspect, traditional yoga classes often provide a sense of community among participants, fostering connections through shared experiences and challenges. Chair yoga, although potentially offered in group settings, might cater to a more diverse group or might be practiced individually at home, which could affect the communal vibe. However, chair yoga classes can also serve as a unique gathering space, especially for people who might feel excluded from more conventional fitness settings.

The comparison between chair yoga and traditional yoga extends to the mental and spiritual benefits as well. True, both practices emphasize the importance of breathwork, meditation, and mindfulness. Yet, the manner in which these elements are taught and experienced can vary. Chair yoga practitioners often highlight the adaptability and practical application of mindfulness and meditation in everyday situations, tailored to their specific lifestyle and capabilities.

Cost and equipment also play a role in evaluating chair yoga against traditional yoga. Generally, chair yoga requires minimal equipment – typically just a sturdy, armless chair. Traditional yoga may necessitate a variety of props, such as yoga mats, blocks, and straps. The simplicity of chair yoga makes it a cost-effective and low-barrier option for beginners or those on a tight budget.

The physical intensity of traditional yoga can be both a pro and a con, depending on an individual's health and fitness level. For some, the challenge of mastering complex poses provides a sense of accomplishment and physical improvement. For others, especially those dealing with physical restrictions, these demands can be discouraging. Chair yoga offers an empowering alternative, emphasizing personal progress and adaptability over competition and comparison.

Another noteworthy difference lies in the practice setting. While traditional yoga often takes place in dedicated studios, chair yoga's versatility allows it to be practiced in various environments, including at home, in the office, or even outdoors. This flexibility not only makes yoga more accessible but also encourages practitioners to incorporate mindfulness and movement into their daily routines in a practical and doable manner.

For those concerned with staying motivated, chair yoga provides an encouraging entry point. The satisfaction of engaging in yoga, perhaps for the first time, can ignite a passion for wellness and a desire to explore further. Meanwhile, traditional yoga practitioners often pursue goals related to mastering specific poses or deepening their practice, which may not resonate with everyone's fitness or health journey.

Injury prevention and management present another crucial consideration. Traditional yoga, if not practiced with proper guidance and attention to bodily limitations, can lead to strain or injury. Chair yoga, designed with safety and accessibility in mind, minimizes these risks, making it an excellent choice for individuals recovering from injury or looking to avoid undue stress on the body.

Ultimately, the choice between chair yoga and traditional yoga should be guided by personal health, goals, and preferences. Chair yoga offers a welcoming, inclusive, and adaptable approach to wellness that meets individuals where they are, both physically and emotionally. It serves as a testament to the universal applicability of yoga principles: mindfulness, flexibility, and strength.

In your journey toward a healthier lifestyle, remember that the most effective exercise is the one you can do consistently and with joy. Chair yoga stands as a powerful testament to the adaptability of yoga, ensuring that its transformative benefits are accessible to all. Embrace the practice that speaks to you, honors your body, and supports your path to wellness.

Benefits Over Other Low-Impact Exercises

When embarking on a journey toward a healthier lifestyle, it's vital to choose a fitness regimen that not only addresses our physical needs but also nurtures our mental and emotional well-being. Chair yoga emerges as a beacon of inclusivity and adaptability in the vast sea of low-impact exercises, offering a unique set of benefits that cater to a broad spectrum of individuals.

Unlike many forms of exercise that require a base level of fitness or mobility, chair yoga is incredibly accessible. It doesn't discriminate based on age, flexibility, or physical condition. This inclusivity is a pivotal advantage, as it opens the doors to health and wellness to those who might feel alienated by more traditional or high-intensity workouts. Imagine transforming an ordinary chair into a tool for health, balance, and rejuvenation - that's the power of chair yoga.

One of the standout benefits of chair yoga, when compared to other low-impact exercises like swimming or walking, is its convenience. You don't need a large space, special equipment, or even good weather - just a chair and a few minutes of your day. This convenience ensures consistency, a key factor in achieving long-term health benefits.

Chair yoga also offers a comprehensive approach to fitness, blending physical movement with breathwork and meditation. This holistic synergy is often missing in other exercises, which may focus solely on physical aspects. By promoting deep breathing and mindfulness, chair yoga helps reduce stress and anxiety, enhancing mental clarity and emotional balance.

For those concerned about joint health, chair yoga presents a gentle yet effective option. The practice minimizes strain on the body's joints, making it an ideal choice for individuals with arthritis or osteoporosis. This contrasts with other low-impact exercises that, while beneficial, may still place some degree of stress on the joints, such as cycling or elliptical training.

Another significant benefit of chair yoga is its adaptability. It can be modified to suit any fitness level, ensuring that everyone, from beginners to seasoned yogis, can participate and benefit. This adaptability also means that as you grow stronger and more flexible, chair yoga grows with you, offering more challenging variations to keep you engaged and progressing.

Flexibility and balance are key components of a healthy body, and chair yoga places a strong emphasis on these elements. By improving these aspects of physical health, chair yoga can reduce the risk of falls and injuries, a consideration particularly important for older adults.

From a postural perspective, chair yoga can work wonders. Many of us suffer from the consequences of a sedentary lifestyle, leading to poor posture and back pain. Chair yoga provides targeted exercises to strengthen core muscles, release tension in the shoulders and neck, and ultimately improve posture.

Chair yoga fosters a community atmosphere, even when practiced alone. There is a vast online community of chair yogis, sharing their journeys and tips. This sense of belonging can motivate you to stay on track and feel supported in your health journey, a motivational boost that is sometimes missing in solitary exercises like jogging or using a stationary bike.

Unlike activities that may spike your heart rate or challenge your endurance, chair yoga places a strong emphasis on nurturing and self-care. It encourages you to listen to your body, to move with intention and respect for your limits. This mindful approach cultivates a deeper connection with your body, teaching valuable lessons in patience and self-acceptance.

The cardiovascular benefits of chair yoga, while gentle, are notable. Through consistent practice, it can help improve circulation and reduce high blood pressure, offering a safe way for those with cardiovascular concerns to exercise and strengthen their heart.

Chair yoga also has the advantage of providing relief from chronic conditions, such as sciatica or fibromyalgia. By focusing on gentle stretching and strengthening, it can alleviate symptoms and improve quality of life for individuals dealing with persistent pain, a feature not always present in other low-impact exercises.

The practice of chair yoga is not just about physical health; it's a gateway to better mental health. The incorporation of meditation and breathwork into the sessions helps combat depression and elevates mood, illustrating how chair yoga touches aspects of well-being that go beyond mere physical fitness.

Lastly, chair yoga's scalability ensures it's a practice that can evolve with technology and research. As we learn more about the human body and wellness, chair yoga adapts, integrating new techniques and approaches to remain at the forefront of accessible health practices. This ability to evolve is something that makes chair yoga not just an exercise, but a lifelong companion in your health journey.

In essence, chair yoga stands out among other low-impact exercises for its unparalleled accessibility, adaptability, and holistic approach to wellness. It encourages individuals to embark on a journey of health that respects the body's limitations while nurturing the mind and spirit. Whether you're seeking to improve flexibility, reduce stress, or simply incorporate more movement into your day, chair yoga offers a pathway to better health that is inviting, effective, and, most importantly, attainable for everyone.

Considering Your Needs and Goals

Embarking on any new exercise regimen, including chair yoga, isn't just about taking the first step; it's about ensuring those steps align with your personal needs and goals. Understanding how chair yoga fits into your lifestyle and what you aim to achieve is paramount. Whether your goal is enhancing flexibility, reducing stress, or improving your overall wellbeing, chair yoga offers a path, but it's essential to navigate this path mindfully.

First, evaluate your physical needs. Chair yoga is renowned for its accessibility and adaptability, making it an excellent choice for those with mobility issues, recovering from injuries, or individuals who spend extensive periods seated. If your aim is to introduce gentle movement into your day, alleviate aches, or enhance your mobility, chair yoga could be the answer you're looking for.

Consider your wellness goals, too. Beyond the physical benefits, chair yoga provides profound mental and emotional advantages. Amidst our fast-paced lives, stress management and mental clarity stand paramount. Chair yoga's incorporation of meditative practices and focused breathing can be a sanctuary for those seeking peace in a turbulent sea of daily pressures.

What about your fitness aspirations? If you're considering chair yoga as part of a broader fitness regimen, it's vital to align it with your overall objectives. While chair yoga can increase flexibility and muscle strength, it's often more gentle than other forms of exercise. However, it can perfectly complement more vigorous workouts by providing necessary recovery and stretching sessions.

Think about the feasibility and sustainability of integrating chair yoga into your daily routine. One of chair yoga's greatest strengths is its convenience. Whether you're a busy professional seeking a quick midday refresh or someone homebound looking for an accessible fitness solution, chair yoga can seamlessly fit into your life. Nonetheless, reflecting on how and when you'll practice is crucial for long-term adherence.

Assess the social and emotional aspects of your wellness journey. Chair yoga, often practiced in groups, can offer a sense of community and support crucial for some. Yet, it's equally effective when practiced solo at home. Identifying whether you thrive in a communal setting or prefer the solitude of a personal practice can guide you toward the right practice environment for your chair yoga journey.

Don't forget to contemplate your learning preferences. Some individuals thrive on in-person instruction, finding it easier to understand the nuances of poses with direct feedback, while others prefer the flexibility and comfort of following online tutorials at their own pace. Consider what learning method resonates with you to enhance your chair yoga experience.

Consideration of personal challenges and limitations is also essential. While chair yoga is adaptable, every person has unique considerations. Whether it's dealing with chronic pain, finding the right chair, or modifying poses to suit your body, understanding these challenges upfront can help tailor your practice to be both beneficial and enjoyable.

Setting clear, realistic goals is a cornerstone of any successful wellness practice. Whether you aim to practice chair yoga daily, increase your flexibility over several months, or simply incorporate more mindfulness into your day, having specific objectives will keep you motivated and provide a barometer for your progress.

Reflect on your reasons for choosing chair yoga over other exercises. It could be the gentleness, the accessibility, or perhaps the holistic approach to wellness that appeals to you. Recognizing what draws you to chair yoga can reinforce your commitment and enhance your practice's enjoyment.

Financial considerations play a role as well. Thankfully, chair yoga can be an extremely cost-effective form of exercise. Unlike many other fitness pursuits, it requires minimal equipment. A sturdy chair and perhaps a few simple props are all that's necessary to begin, making it an accessible option for those on a tight budget.

Given chair yoga's versatility, it can cater to a broad spectrum of individuals and intentions. Whether you're a senior looking to maintain mobility, a desk-bound professional aiming to negate the effects of prolonged sitting, or simply someone seeking a gentle entry point into fitness, chair yoga can be tailored to meet those needs.

However, like any form of exercise, the benefits of chair yoga are most pronounced with regular practice. Consistency is key. Establishing a routine, even if it's just a few minutes a day, can lead to significant improvements over time. Embrace the journey with patience, understanding that the rewards will unfold as you progress.

While chair yoga offers numerous benefits and can be a perfect fit for many, it's also important to listen to your body and respond to its feedback. If certain poses cause discomfort, or if you find aspects of the practice don't meet your needs, don't hesitate to adapt. Remember, the ultimate goal is your health and wellbeing.

In summary, considering your needs and goals in the context of chair yoga requires a holistic approach. It's about pinpointing what you seek to achieve, understanding the unique benefits chair yoga can offer, and fitting this approach into your life in a way that feels natural and fulfilling. With thoughtful consideration and regular practice, chair yoga can be a profoundly impactful part of your wellness journey.

Chapter 9:
Enhancing Your Practice With Props
and Modifications

As we delve into the world of Chair Yoga, it's essential to recognize that our practices can be significantly amplified by the strategic use of props and modifications. This chapter aims to demystify the notion that props signify a lesser practice. On the contrary, they are the unsung heroes that make yoga truly accessible and tailored to each individual's needs. Whether it's using a strap to extend your reach or a block to ground your posture, these tools are here to support and challenge your body, guiding you towards a deeper understanding of each pose.

But it's not just about what props you use; it's how you use them. Here, we'll navigate through common poses, offering creative and safe ways to modify them. This ensures that no matter your level of mobility or strength, the transformative power of yoga remains within your grasp. Additionally, moving through each modification, you'll discover that the real strength lies in honoring your body's unique needs at any given moment.

To practice safely is to practice with mindfulness. As we explore the treasure trove of props and pose adaptations, you'll learn tips to keep your practice not only effective but also safe. This mindful approach ensures that your journey with chair yoga is not just about the physicality but also about fostering a symbiotic relationship between body, mind, and spirit. So, let's embark on this journey together, where each prop becomes a stepping stone toward achieving a healthier lifestyle, affirming that yoga, with its infinite adaptability, truly is for everyone.

Using Props for Support and Challenge

When embarking on a journey of health and flexibility, it's crucial to recognize that the tools we choose can significantly enhance our practice. In the realm of chair yoga, props aren't merely accessories; they are allies in our quest for a healthier lifestyle. Embracing props offers both support and challenge, enabling practitioners to deepen their practice in ways they never thought possible.

Props, including blocks, straps, and even the chair itself, provide a foundation to explore poses with greater alignment and safety. For beginners, this means an opportunity to engage in poses with the correct form, minimizing the risk of injury. For the seasoned practitioner, props invite an exploration of depth and endurance in familiar poses, presenting a fresh challenge and furthering the journey of flexibility and strength.

Consider the block, often viewed merely as a tool for support. When strategically placed, a block can elevate the hips in a seated forward bend, offering an extended range of motion and a deeper stretch. Conversely, for those seeking to challenge their balance and strength, a block can serve as a precarious perch for the feet in poses such as the chair pigeon, demanding finer control and increased focus.

Straps, likewise, aren't just for those who can't touch their toes. They serve as an extension of the arms, enabling practitioners to grasp legs, feet, or even pull against for enhanced stretching and opening of the body. By adjusting the length and tension of the strap, one can modulate the level of challenge in a pose, exploring the edges of their flexibility and strength in a controlled manner.

The chair, the central prop in chair yoga, is a versatile tool. Beyond serving as a seat, it can transform into a support for standing poses, offering a handhold for balance or a brace for stretching. Yet, this same tool can become a challenge by demanding more from one's balance and coordination in poses such as the standing mountain pose, where hands might reach high above the chair, or in a twisted chair pose that requires maintaining balance while turning the torso.

Incorporating props into your chair yoga practice isn't just about making poses accessible or more challenging; it's about listening to your body and respecting its needs and limits. Props allow for modifications that can help avoid strain in areas of sensitivity, such as the lower back or knees, ensuring a practice that is not only beneficial but sustainable.

More than physical supports, props also embody the principle of mindfulness. They remind us to be present, to pay attention to the alignment of our bodies, and to practice with intention. Every prop used is a cue to engage fully with the practice, to connect mind, body, and breath in a harmonious flow.

Yet, it's important to remember that the use of props is a personal choice, reflective of one's journey and goals in yoga. Whether you're using a prop to deepen a stretch, to find greater stability, or to experiment with new poses, what matters most is that it serves your practice. Encourage exploration and adjustment, and remain open to the possibilities that props can introduce to your chair yoga experience.

Adopting props into your practice also fosters creativity. Imagine using a strap not just for stretching but as a tool for resistance exercises, or leveraging the chair for inverted poses where the legs are elevated, promoting circulation. The possibilities are limited only by your imagination and willingness to experiment.

For those intimidated by the use of props, start simple. Integrate one prop at a time, allowing yourself to become accustomed to its feel and function. Observe how its inclusion alters your practice, noting any shifts in ease, comfort, or challenge. Remember, there is no rush in the journey of self-discovery and health.

Documentation of your progress can be enlightening. Keep a practice journal, noting which props were used and how they influenced your experience of different poses. This not only serves as a personal record but as a motivational tool, showcasing how far you've come and the various ways you've adapted your practice to meet your evolving needs.

Moreover, props are a testament to the evolution of yoga as a practice that is inclusive and adaptable. They signify a shift from a one-size-fits-all approach to a recognition of the unique paths we all walk in our journey toward health and well-being. Whether it's through supporting a healing injury or challenging a seasoned yogi to deepen their practice, props are invaluable tools in the pursuit of personal growth and self-awareness.

In conclusion, the strategic use of props in chair yoga can transform your practice from a routine exercise into a profound exploration of self. They offer support, introduce challenge, and encourage a deeper connection with the inner workings of one's body and mind. So, as you continue on your path toward a healthier lifestyle, let props be your companions, guiding you towards greater strength, flexibility, and mindfulness.

Embrace the journey with an open heart and mind, and let the world of chair yoga with props open up new horizons in your quest for health. Remember, the goal is not to perfect a pose but to find balance and harmony within yourself. With each prop and pose, you're not just enhancing your practice; you're expanding the boundaries of what you thought possible, embarking on a journey of discovery, one pose at a time.

Modifications for Common Poses

As we explore the journey of chair yoga together, it's essential to recognize that not every pose will fit every body exactly the same way. And that's perfectly okay. Just like life, yoga is about finding what works for you and adapting as necessary. The beauty of chair yoga lies in its flexibility and the ability to modify common poses to suit your needs, enhancing your practice and ensuring it remains both safe and effective.

Let's start with the Seated Forward Bend, a staple in the flexibility and balance category of poses. If reaching for your toes feels like a distant dream, consider placing a cushion or yoga block on top of your feet. This simple modification decreases the distance you need to stretch, allowing you to experience the pose's benefits without straining.

Moving on to the Chair Pigeon, which can be quite challenging for those with tight hips. A fantastic modification involves simply crossing your ankle over the opposite knee, creating a figure-four shape. Focus on keeping your spine long and pushing gently on the knee of the crossed leg to deepen the stretch according to your comfort level.

Another common pose is the Chair Cat-Cow, which is excellent for spinal flexibility. If you find the arching and rounding of the back uncomfortable, consider reducing the range of motion. Instead of focusing on how deep the bend is, concentrate on the movement's fluidity and the stretching sensation along your spine.

The Chair Warrior poses are another area where modifications can be highly beneficial. If maintaining balance while transitioning between Warrior I and II poses is challenging, keep your feet closer together. This adjustment provides more stability while still strengthening your legs and improving flexibility.

For those who find the Chair Twist poses difficult due to back issues or limited mobility, you can modify by reducing the twist range. Instead of aiming for a complete rotation, focus on turning from your waist just to the point where you can feel the stretch without any discomfort.

In Chair Yoga, props are not just tools; they are extensions of the practice itself. For instance, in poses that involve reaching towards the floor, like a modified Standing Forward Bend using the chair for support, blocks can be placed on the ground to "bring the floor closer" to you.

Then there's the Seated Mountain Pose, which seems straightforward but can be quite challenging in maintaining the elongation of the spine. Here, a small folded towel or blanket placed under your sitting bones can help tilt your pelvis slightly forward, making it easier to sit up straight.

Let's not forget about the breathing techniques integral to yoga practice. If deep, seated breaths are challenging, try sitting at the edge of the chair to allow your diaphragm more space. This subtle shift can significantly impact your ability to breathe deeply and fully.

For those working on improving balance through Chair Yoga, props like a wall or a sturdy table can be immensely helpful. Use them for support in poses like the Chair Tree Pose, where balance can be a significant challenge. Over time, you might find yourself relying less on these supports as your strength and confidence grow.

When engaging in meditative practices or longer-held poses, comfort is key. A cushion or folded blanket on the chair for seated poses or under the knees for poses practiced while lying down can make a significant difference. Comfort in practice encourages longer, deeper engagement with meditation and relaxation poses.

Adapting practices for specific needs is not just about personal comfort; it's about ensuring that yoga remains inclusive and accessible. Chair Yoga embodies this by allowing each individual to tailor their practice. If a pose doesn't feel right, listen to your body and adjust as necessary. This responsiveness to your body's needs is at the heart of mindfulness.

Finally, remember that the alignment of poses is more about how it feels than how it looks. In Chair Yoga, the aim is not to achieve the perfect form but to connect with your body and breath in a way that feels nurturing and beneficial to you.

Incorporating these modifications into your chair yoga practice can significantly enhance not only the physical benefits you receive but also your connection to the practice. Each modification serves as a reminder that yoga is a personal journey, one that respects and celebrates individual differences and needs.

As you continue to explore chair yoga, embrace the opportunity to customize your practice. This personalization not only fosters a deeper connection to your yoga journey but also supports a healthy, balanced life. The path to wellness is unique for everyone, and chair yoga, with its adaptable nature, offers a beautiful, inclusive way to walk this path. So, keep experimenting, adjusting, and finding what feels right for you. Your practice, your way.

Tips for Safe Practice

The journey toward enhancing your chair yoga practice is both exhilarating and transformative. However, ensuring safety during your practice is paramount. As we explore the array of props and modifications available, remember, the primary goal is to cultivate a practice that honors your body's unique needs and limitations without compromising your wellbeing. Let's dive into some vital tips to keep your practice both safe and impactful.

First and foremost, selecting the right chair is crucial. Ensure your chair is sturdy and doesn't have wheels. If it happens to have wheels, secure them against movement. A stable foundation is the bedrock of a safe chair yoga practice, enabling you to explore poses with confidence and ease.

When introducing props into your practice, start with the basics like blocks and straps. These can enhance your poses by bringing the ground closer or aiding in reaching further. However, always ensure that any prop used is applied in a manner that supports rather than strains. A prop should never push you beyond your comfortable range of motion.

Modifications are not merely alternatives; they are intelligent adaptations that respect your body's capability on any given day. Embrace them wholeheartedly. For instance, if a pose suggests lifting your arms high but your shoulders feel tight, consider a modification where you keep your hands resting on your lap. Respect your body's limits.

Consistency is key, but so is listening to your body. Some days you might feel more flexible or strong, and on other days, you might need to take it easy. Adjust your practice accordingly. Pushing through pain is not a badge of honor; it's a risk to your health.

Be mindful of transitions between poses. Move slowly and deliberately, especially when moving in and out of poses that challenge your balance or require a significant shift in weight distribution. Rushed movements can compromise stability and increase the risk of injury.

Invest time in warming up at the beginning of your practice. Gentle movements and mindful breathing help to prepare your body and mind, reducing the risk of strain. Similarly, cooling down is just as important to gradually lower your heart rate and signal to your body that the practice is coming to an end.

Focus on alignment, even in a seemingly simple pose. Proper alignment ensures optimal benefits from each pose while safeguarding against undue stress on joints and muscles. If unsure about the correct alignment, seek guidance from a knowledgeable instructor or trusted resources.

Hydration is often overlooked in the context of yoga practice. However, keeping your body adequately hydrated is essential for maintaining flexibility and preventing cramps.

Make sure to drink water before and after your practice, and listen to your body's hydration cues.

Pay attention to your breath. It's not just a vital component of your practice; it's a guide. If your breathing becomes strained or erratic, it might be an indicator that you're pushing too hard. Allow your breath to guide the intensity of your practice.

Remember, yoga is not a competition. The journey is personal and subjective. Avoid comparing your practice or progress to others'. Focus on your own path, celebrating your achievements and acknowledging areas for growth without judgment.

Incorporate restorative poses into your practice, especially if you've been challenging your body with more strenuous poses. Poses like a seated forward bend can offer a soothing counteraction, promoting relaxation and recovery.

If practicing chair yoga to address or manage specific health concerns, consult with a healthcare provider to tailor your practice appropriately. This is especially important for individuals with chronic conditions or injuries. A collaborative approach ensures that your practice supports your health goals.

Finally, cultivate patience and kindness toward yourself. Progress in yoga isn't linear, and every practice offers a new opportunity to learn and grow. Celebrate where you are at this moment, and trust in the journey ahead.

By adhering to these tips, your chair yoga practice will not only be safer but also more enjoyable and fulfilling. Embrace the process of learning and growing, using your practice as a compass guiding you toward greater health, flexibility, and well-being.

Chapter 10:
Nutrition and Wellness for Chair Yogis

Embarking on the journey of chair yoga, we now turn the spotlight to a vital component that fuels our practice: nutrition. For chair yogis, understanding and integrating the principles of nutrition and wellness into their routine can significantly amplify the benefits of their practice. It's about creating a synergy between what we do on the chair and how we nourish our bodies off it. Think of your body as a garden; just as the right balance of sunlight, water, and soil nurtures plants, a balanced diet energizes and revitalizes your body, enhancing flexibility, strength, and mental clarity.

Nutrition doesn't have to be complex or restrictive. Simple dietary adjustments, focusing on whole foods, can make a profound difference. Incorporate a rainbow of fruits and vegetables, lean proteins, whole grains, and healthy fats to supply your body with an array of nutrients essential for recovery and energy. This chapter isn't just about what to eat; it's about developing a mindful eating practice, linking the awareness and presence we cultivate in chair yoga to how and why we eat. Imagine eating with the same intention and focus as you bring to your yoga practice—this approach will not only transform your relationship with food but also support your overall wellness journey.

Remember, your path to wellness through chair yoga is holistic, encompassing both the physical movements and the sustenance you provide your body. Whether you're looking to enhance your energy levels, improve digestive health, or simply feel more aligned—nutrition is your foundational support. Let's dive into how you can adopt a mindful eating practice, understand the impact of various foods on your body and spirit, and make nutrition an integral part of your yoga journey. Remember, each small step towards better nutrition is a leap towards amplifying the transformative power of chair yoga.

The Role of Nutrition in Your Yoga Practice

Nutrition plays a critical role in enhancing your yoga journey, particularly in the domain of chair yoga. When you align your eating habits with your physical activities, such as yoga, you're not just working on your flexibility and strength but also nourishing your body in a way that supports both your physical and mental well-being. Balancing the nutrients you consume can significantly affect your energy levels, recovery, and overall yoga experience.

Understanding the connection between the food you eat and your body's performance is the first step towards integrating nutrition into your yoga practice effectively. Various nutrients contribute to muscle repair, joint health, and metabolic efficiency, which are vital for anyone practicing yoga, including chair yogis. Every morsel of food you ingest can either fuel your practice or hinder it, depending on your choices.

Protein, for example, is essential for muscle repair. Incorporating a moderate amount of lean protein into your diet can help rebuild the muscles that you're engaging during your chair yoga sessions. This doesn't mean you need to consume large quantities of meat or protein shakes; plant-based sources like lentils, beans, and tofu are excellent options that fit well into a yogic diet.

Hydration is another critical aspect that tends to be overlooked. Water aids in almost every function of the body, including the flexibility of muscles and joints. Staying adequately hydrated will make a noticeable difference in your yoga practice, making poses easier and more fluid. Additionally, incorporating herbal teas can also provide hydration while introducing antioxidants that support overall health.

Carbohydrates are the body's primary energy source. Choosing complex carbohydrates such as whole grains, fruits, and vegetables instead of refined sugars provides a steady energy release. This sustained energy is particularly beneficial during longer yoga sessions, helping to maintain focus and stamina from start to finish.

Fats, often misunderstood and wrongly vilified, are crucial for long-term energy, cell growth, and the absorption of certain vitamins. Including healthy fats from sources like avocados, nuts, and seeds in your diet supports your body's wellness and aids in the overall yoga experience.

Speaking of vitamins and minerals, they play vital roles in ensuring that the body's systems operate smoothly. For instance, calcium and magnesium are important for bone health and muscle function—two elements heavily involved in yoga. Iron, which helps transport oxygen throughout the body, is crucial for maintaining energy levels during physical activity.

An often-overlooked component of nutrition as it relates to yoga is timing. Consuming a heavy meal just before your practice can lead to discomfort, while practicing on an empty stomach might leave you feeling weak and distracted by hunger. Finding a balance by eating a light, nourishing snack an hour or so before your session can provide the energy you need without the discomfort.

Listening to your body is paramount. It's easy to get bogged down by specific dietary guidelines, but everyone's body reacts differently to foods. Some might find that a small piece of fruit provides the perfect pre-yoga boost, while others may prefer a handful of nuts. Observing how different foods affect your energy and comfort during yoga will guide you to the best choices for your body.

Integrating mindful eating practices with your yoga routine can amplify the benefits of both. Mindful eating involves paying full attention to the experience of eating and drinking, both inside and outside the body. It encourages an awareness of the physical and sensual cues associated with eating, which can lead to a more harmonious relationship with food, akin to the harmony sought through yoga.

Seasonality is another aspect worthy of attention. Eating foods that are in season aligns with the yoga principle of living in harmony with nature. Seasonal fruits and vegetables not only taste better but are also at their nutritional peak. This practice supports local farmers and minimizes the environmental impact, reflecting the yogic principle of Ahimsa, or non-harm.

A common misconception is that following a nutritional plan that supports your yoga practice must be restrictive. On the contrary, it's about making choices that nourish your body and enhance your practice. Rather than focusing on what you shouldn't eat, concentrate on the abundance of foods that can help you feel your best—both on and off the chair.

Finally, remember that changes to your diet should be implemented gradually. Drastic changes can lead to discomfort and resistance, whereas small, manageable adjustments are more likely to become sustainable habits. Just as chair yoga is about meeting your body where it's at, so too is nutritional wellness.

By embracing a holistic approach to nutrition and wellness, chair yogis can greatly enhance their practice and overall well-being. Through mindful selection, preparation, and consumption of food, one can support their physical yoga practice while promoting mental clarity and emotional balance. This harmonious blend of nutrition and yoga creates a solid foundation for a vibrant, healthy life.

In conclusion, the integration of nutrition into your yoga practice is not just about enhancing physical performance; it's about nurturing your body, respecting its needs, and fostering a deep, sustaining connection between the food you eat and your spiritual and physical yoga journey. Embrace this relationship with an open mind and heart, and watch as your practice—and your life—transforms.

Simple Dietary Adjustments for Better Health

Embarking on a journey towards better health doesn't have to mean overhauling your entire lifestyle overnight. In fact, some of the most significant strides toward wellness can start with small, simple dietary adjustments. Nutrition plays a crucial role in supporting your chair yoga practice and enhancing overall well-being. This section will guide you through practical and manageable changes you can make to your diet that align with your path to health and flexibility.

First and foremost, hydration is key. Often, we underestimate the power of drinking enough water throughout the day. Every cell in your body needs water to function properly. Begin by increasing your water intake gradually. Aim to add an extra glass of water to your daily routine each week until you reach the recommended eight glasses a day. If plain water doesn't excite you, infuse it with fruits or herbs like strawberries, cucumber, or mint for a refreshing twist.

Next, let's talk vegetables. Increasing your vegetable intake can have profound effects on your health, providing essential nutrients and fiber. But don't worry; you don't have to suddenly start consuming salads at every meal. Small steps, such as adding a handful of spinach to your morning smoothie or snacking on baby carrots, can significantly contribute to your vegetable intake. Remember, it's about progression, not perfection.

Another adjustment is to slowly shift towards whole grains. If you're accustomed to white bread or pasta, start by mixing in their whole-grain counterparts until you've fully transitioned. Whole grains contain more nutrients and fiber, supporting digestion and providing a steady energy release, which is essential during your chair yoga sessions.

Sugar is a tricky beast. Reducing added sugars in your diet can dramatically improve your health, but it's a challenging habit to break. Begin by noticing where added sugars show up in your diet—often in places you might not expect, like salad dressings or bread. Gradually decrease your consumption of these items, and opt for natural sweeteners like fruit, or a small amount of honey or maple syrup when you need a sweet fix.

Lean proteins are essential, especially if you're engaging in any form of exercise, including chair yoga. Incorporating a variety of protein sources, such as beans, lentils, fish, lean meats, or tofu, can support muscle repair and growth. If you're not used to eating much protein, start by adding a small portion to one meal a day and increase from there as your body adjusts.

Don't forget about healthy fats. Not all fats are created equal, and your body needs certain fats for energy and to support cell growth. Add avocado to your toast, snack on a handful of nuts, or cook with olive oil to ensure you're getting a good balance of healthy fats.

Balancing your meals is also crucial. Start thinking of your plate in portions: half filled with vegetables, a quarter with lean protein, and a quarter with whole grains or healthy starches. This balance can help ensure you're getting a mix of essential nutrients at each meal.

Limiting processed foods is another step toward better health. Processed foods can be convenient, but they're often filled with unhealthy fats, added sugars, and sodium. Begin by identifying one processed item you can do without, and eliminate it from your diet. Gradually, continue to find alternatives for processed foods until your diet consists more of whole, unprocessed foods.

Snacking smart is also vital. Instead of reaching for chips or cookies, prep healthy snacks like sliced veggies and hummus, fruit, or a small portion of nuts. These snacks can provide energy without the sugar crash, supporting your overall wellness and yoga practice.

Mindful eating is a practice that perfectly complements chair yoga. It involves paying full attention to the experience of eating and drinking, both inside and outside the body. Notice the colors, smells, textures, and flavors of your food, and listen to your body's hunger and fullness signals. This practice can help reduce overeating and increase satisfaction with your meals.

Consider the timing of your meals too. Eating your meals and snacks at roughly the same time each day can help regulate your body's hunger cues and support better digestion and energy levels. It's especially beneficial to have a light snack or meal a couple of hours before your chair yoga session to ensure you have the energy to participate fully.

Lastly, remember that these changes don't have to happen all at once. It's about making small adjustments over time. Celebrate your victories, no matter how small, and be kind to yourself during setbacks. Progress, not perfection, is the goal.

Incorporating these simple dietary adjustments into your routine can significantly impact your health and wellness, complementing your chair yoga practice. Each small change you make is a step towards a healthier, more vibrant you. Embrace these adjustments with an open heart and mind, and watch as your body responds positively, supporting you in your journey to better health through chair yoga and beyond.

Remember, every journey starts with a single step—or in this case, a single dietary adjustment. Choose one or two adjustments to begin with, and gradually build from there. With each positive change, you'll not only feel better physically but you'll also strengthen your commitment to a healthier, more mindful lifestyle—a cornerstone of the chair yoga philosophy.

Linking Mindful Eating with Yoga Principles

Yoga isn't just about stretching or holding poses. It's a lifestyle that encompasses how we treat our bodies, how we breathe, and yes, even how we eat. Turning our attention to the principles of mindful eating, we see a beautiful synergy with the essence of yoga. The practice of becoming more in tune with our bodies, our needs, and the moment itself isn't restricted to the mat—it extends to the dining table too.

At its heart, mindful eating is about awareness. Just as yoga teaches us to be present in each pose, mindful eating urges us to focus on every bite. It invites us to savor our food, to chew slowly, and to appreciate the flavors, textures, and aromas. This process turns each meal into a meditative experience, allowing us to connect with the present and listen to the cues our bodies are giving us about hunger and satisfaction.

Another core yoga principle is ahimsa, or non-harm, which naturally aligns with mindful eating. This approach encourages us to make dietary choices that not only nourish our bodies but also cause the least harm to other beings and the planet. It prompts us to consider where our food comes from, how it was produced, and its impact on the environment.

Satya, or truthfulness, compels us to be honest with ourselves about why we eat what we eat. Are we reaching for nutritious foods that genuinely nourish our bodies, or are we indulging in comfort food to cope with emotional stress? Yoga inspires a search for truth in all aspects of our lives, including our eating habits.

The principle of saucha, or cleanliness, resonates through yoga and mindful eating as well. A clean diet, consisting of fresh, whole foods, mirrors the internal cleanliness we strive for in our yoga practice. This doesn't mean we need to follow a strict diet but rather choose foods that make us feel vibrant and alive.

Brahmacharya, often interpreted as moderation, teaches us balance. Just as we seek equilibrium in our yoga poses, in mindful eating, we look for a balanced approach to what and how much we consume. This principle helps us avoid overindulgence and honor our body's genuine needs.

Aparigraha, or non-attachment, invites us to let go of our emotional dependencies on food. Instead of relying on food for comfort or distraction, we learn to appreciate it as nourishment. This doesn't mean we can't enjoy our meals, but rather that we don't allow our happiness to depend solely on them.

Integrating these yoga principles into our eating habits can transform meals into a rich, fulfilling experience. This approach encourages us to eat mindfully, choosing foods that benefit both our bodies and the broader world. Silencing the distractions and truly listening to what our bodies need may take practice, but the benefits are immense.

Start by paying attention to the sensations that arise as you eat. Notice the textures and flavors of your food, the thoughts and emotions that surface. Are you eating because you're truly hungry, or are there other factors at play?

Embrace gratitude for your meal. Before eating, take a moment to reflect on the journey your food has taken to reach your plate. This can deepen your connection to the earth and its cycles, fostering a sense of interconnectedness that is central to yoga philosophy.

Experiment with creating a serene, distraction-free dining environment. Just as a calm and dedicated space enhances your yoga practice, a peaceful eating setting can help reinforce your mindful eating habits.

Challenge yourself to make one change at a time. Perhaps you start by choosing one meal a day to eat mindfully, free from distractions like screens or books. Gradually, as this practice becomes a habit, you might find yourself naturally making healthier food choices that align with your body's needs.

Remember, the aim isn't perfection but progress. It's about making incremental changes that benefit your physical and mental well-being. Just as each yoga session is an opportunity for growth, each meal is a chance to practice mindfulness and nourish your body in a way that honors its needs.

Linking mindful eating with yoga principles offers a holistic approach to health that celebrates the unity of body, mind, and spirit. It's an invitation to slow down, to be present, and to cultivate a deeper respect for the food we eat and the bodies we nourish. As chair yogis, embracing these practices can enhance our wellness journey, making each meal a reflective and enriching extension of our yoga practice.

As we continue to explore the vast world of yoga, incorporating mindful eating into our lifestyle is a powerful step towards harmonizing our internal and external worlds. It's an opportunity to embody the principles of yoga, not just on the mat, but in every aspect of our lives, including the way we eat. So let's approach our meals with the same intention and gratitude we bring to our yoga practice, transforming them into yet another path toward health, joy, and balance.

Chapter 11:
Stories of Transformation

In this inspiring chapter, we dive into the heartwarming and invigorating stories of individuals who found a new lease on life through chair yoga. These narratives aren't just testimonials; they're a testament to the resilience of the human spirit and the transformative power of incorporating mindful movement and breathing into one's routine. From folks who faced mobility challenges to those wrestling with stress and its myriad effects, chair yoga has emerged as a beacon of hope, guiding them towards a healthier, more fulfilling lifestyle. Each story unfolds to reveal personal journeys of overcoming obstacles, finding inner strength, and achieving a sense of balance and wellness that once seemed out of reach. As we explore these compelling accounts, you'll see chair yoga not just as a series of poses, but as a pathway to reclaiming one's health and vitality. It's these stories that illuminate the profound impact chair yoga can have on the body, mind, and soul, encouraging anyone, regardless of their starting point, to embark on their own journey of transformation.

Mike Ezekiel

Real-Life Success Stories

In the world of wellness and transformation, the power of personal stories cannot be overstated. Each narrative is a testament to the resilience of the human spirit, and the journey through chair yoga is no exception. These real-life accounts not only inspire but also provide a road map for those on the path to a healthier lifestyle. Let's dive into the lives of individuals who have experienced remarkable transformations through chair yoga.

Emma, a 58-year-old with chronic arthritis, felt her world shrinking as her mobility decreased. The pain made it hard for her to engage in activities she loved, and she feared the isolation that might come with it. That was until she discovered chair yoga. Initially skeptical, Emma found the gentle poses accessible and noticed a reduction in her pain levels after just a few sessions. Months into her practice, she has regained mobility in her joints and now leads a more active and joyful life.

John's story is equally compelling. After a car accident left him with persistent lower back pain, the 43-year-old graphic designer saw his ability to sit at a desk diminish. Determined not to let this setback define his career, John turned to chair yoga. The targeted stretches not only alleviated his back pain but also improved his posture, making long hours at the desk more manageable. John credits chair yoga for not just physical relief but a newfound mental resilience against the challenges of recovery.

For 27-year-old Mia, chair yoga was a gateway to managing her anxiety. The fast-paced nature of her job in digital marketing often left her feeling overwhelmed. The breathing exercises and meditative aspects of chair yoga brought her a sense of calm she hadn't experienced in years. It became her daily ritual, transforming not just her mind but influencing her approach to work and personal life with a newfound serenity.

Linda, a retired school teacher, found chair yoga to be the perfect antidote to the loneliness that sometimes accompanied her retirement. The communal aspect of joining a chair yoga class at her local community center gave her a sense of belonging and purpose. The physical benefits were a bonus to the friendships she developed, proving that wellness is a holistic concept that encompasses social connections.

Michael's journey underscores the versatility of chair yoga as a practice. Suffering from obesity, Michael felt intimidated by conventional exercise routines. The inclusivity and adaptability of chair yoga allowed him to start exercising at his own pace. Over time, not only did he lose weight, but he also discovered a passion for nutrition, leading him to make healthier lifestyle choices overall.

These stories highlight but a few of the countless lives touched by the power of chair yoga. From increasing mobility and reducing pain to enhancing mental health and fostering community, the benefits extend far beyond the chair. It's a reminder that transformation is within reach, regardless of where you start. The key is to begin, to take that first step toward a healthier, more vibrant you.

What's remarkable about chair yoga isn't just its accessibility; it's the ripple effect it creates in every aspect of one's life. As seen through these stories, individuals not only see improvements in their physical health but experience profound changes in their mental and emotional well-being. This holistic approach to fitness is what sets chair yoga apart, making it not just a form of exercise, but a lifestyle change that encourages a harmonious balance between body and mind.

The narratives of Emma, John, Mia, Linda, and Michael serve as powerful reminders that change is possible, and it often starts with a small step. A chair and a willingness to transform are all you need to embark on this journey. Whether you're dealing with physical limitations, stress, or looking for a sense of community, chair yoga offers a path towards achieving those goals.

As we reflect on these stories, we're reminded of the importance of an open heart and mind when approaching any form of transformation. The success of these individuals stems not only from their regular practice of chair yoga but also from their belief in the possibility of change. It's this combination of perseverance, faith, and the supportive framework of chair yoga that paves the way for remarkable transformations.

In the end, the journey of health and wellness is deeply personal, yet universally connected by shared experiences. These stories of transformation through chair yoga shine a light on the vast potential within each of us to rehabilitate, rejuvenate, and reconnect with our best selves. As we move forward, let these narratives inspire us to make choices that align with our wellness goals, reminding us that every day is an opportunity to transform and thrive.

How Chair Yoga Changed Lives

Embarking on a journey towards health and flexibility, we've explored the fundamentals, debunked myths, and delved deep into the heart of chair yoga. Now, let's pivot our focus towards the transformative stories that underscore the profound impact chair yoga has made on individuals from various walks of life. These narratives not only serve as a testament to the power of persistence but also illuminate the path for others seeking a similar metamorphosis.

Imagine a world where the limitations of one's body don't dictate the boundaries of one's spirit. This is the world that chair yoga invites us into. Through the lens of those who've embraced this practice, we witness a remarkable unleashing of potential, a rekindling of hope, and a rejuvenation of both body and mind.

Take Sarah, for instance, a 65-year-old retiree who believed her days of physical activity were well behind her due to chronic knee pain. The introduction to chair yoga via a local community center presented a new lease on life. "It was like finding the missing piece of a puzzle," Sarah recounts. Her story is not unique but rather a echo of many who've discovered chair yoga as a gateway to improved mobility and pain management.

Then there's Michael, a middle-aged man grappling with the stressors of a high-pressure job and a sedentary lifestyle.

The concept of yoga seemed foreign, inaccessible, and frankly, not something he pictured himself doing. Chair yoga changed all that. It offered a practical, relatable approach that fit seamlessly into his hectic schedule. The benefits were immediate - better posture, reduced stress, and an overall sense of well-being. Michael's journey highlights the versatility of chair yoga in adapting to the needs of its practitioners.

For someone like Jenna, a young adult with a congenital heart condition, the whispers of limitation had been a constant companion. Yet, chair yoga offered a symphony of empowerment, allowing her to engage in physical activity without overexertion. Her story is a powerful reminder of the adaptability of chair yoga, making it an inclusive practice for those with specific health conditions.

As these stories unfold, a common theme emerges: transformation is not only about the physical changes but the mental and emotional rebirths. The practice of chair yoga transcends the chair itself; it becomes a metaphor for overcoming the restrictions we often place on ourselves or accept from the world around us.

It's not merely the poses that create change, but the breathing techniques and meditation practices that accompany them. They act as tools for managing anxiety, fostering a deep-seated tranquility, and enhancing one's overall mental health.

Moreover, the sense of community found in chair yoga classes plays a pivotal role in these transformations. Sharing space and energy with others on similar journeys fosters a sense of belonging and encouragement. It's in these communal gatherings that individuals find not only accountability but a shared joy in each other's progress.

Indeed, the beauty of chair yoga lies in its accessibility. Whether it's practiced in a studio, at home, or even in the office, it seamlessly integrates into daily routines, proving that the path to wellness need not be arduous but instead can be adapted to fit the contours of one's life.

The versatility of chair yoga is further demonstrated in how it accommodates varying levels of mobility and fitness. From those recovering from surgery to seasoned athletes seeking a gentle practice on rest days, chair yoga meets each individual where they are, embodying true inclusivity.

Importantly, the narratives of those whose lives have been touched by chair yoga dispel the myths that may deter some from embarking on this journey. The misconception that yoga requires a certain level of flexibility or that it's reserved for the young and fit is dismantled story by story, pose by pose.

This transformative journey also extends to nutrition and overall wellness. Many who practice chair yoga become more attuned to their bodies' needs, adopting healthier eating habits and a mindful approach to nutrition. This holistic transformation underscores the interconnectedness of physical activity, mental health, and nutrition.

As we delve into these stories of transformation, we're reminded of the resilience of the human spirit and the capacity for renewal. Chair yoga, with its adaptability and accessibility, serves as a beacon of hope for those searching for a path to better health and flexibility.

Each story is a stepping stone for someone else considering this path. The narratives of Sarah, Michael, Jenna, and countless others serve not only as testimonials of the power of chair yoga but also as invitations to explore a practice that has the potential to redefine lives.

In embracing chair yoga, individuals across the globe are finding a practice that respects their body's limits while challenging them to explore new horizons within themselves. They're discovering that the chair is not a symbol of restriction but a tool of liberation.

In concluding this section, it's clear that chair yoga is more than a physical practice; it's a journey of self-discovery, healing, and transformation. It's an affirmation that regardless of age, mobility, or fitness level, everyone has the potential to achieve greater health and flexibility. The stories shared here are but a few of many, each painting a vivid picture of the transformative power of chair yoga.

Chapter 12:
Teaching Chair Yoga

Entering the realm of teaching chair yoga embodies a remarkable journey, not just for you, but for every individual you guide. This chapter hones in on transforming your passion for chair yoga into a powerful tool for wellness, capable of reaching out and positively affecting lives. Embrace the role of a beacon, guiding individuals through their health and flexibility voyages with chair yoga. Here, we delve into expert guidelines tailored for instructors, covering the spectrum from adapting practices for diverse audiences to fostering a nurturing community for practitioners. It's about grasping the gentle balance between teaching and learning, where every class is a shared experience brimming with growth and discovery.

Start by understanding that everyone's yoga pathway is as unique as their fingerprint. As a teacher, your adaptability and sensitivity to individual needs are paramount. You'll find strategies for tailoring sessions that respect and challenge each person's limits, ensuring a safe yet fulfilling practice. We're not just focusing on the asanas; it's also about igniting a flame of self-awareness and harmony within the mind and body. Cultivating a community around chair yoga transforms this solitary practice into a shared journey, emboldening participants to support and inspire one another.

Your mission is clear. With each pose you demonstrate and every breath you coordinate, you're not only teaching chair yoga; you're also spreading a message of empowerment and resilience. This chapter gives you the tools and insights to bridge gaps, break barriers, and light up that spark of passion for health and wellness in others. Remember, in the grand tapestry of chair yoga, you're not just an instructor. You're a storyteller, a guide, and most importantly, a catalyst for change.

Guidelines for Teachers

Entering the world of teaching chair yoga is an exciting journey that will not only transform the lives of your students but will also deepen your own practice and understanding of yoga. As an instructor, you are tasked with creating a safe, inclusive, and motivating environment that caters to the varied needs of your students. Here, we'll delve into essential guidelines to help you navigate this rewarding path.

First and foremost, it's critical to foster an atmosphere of acceptance and respect in your classes. Remember that participants come from diverse backgrounds and have different physical abilities. As such, it's vital to practice patience and encourage your students to listen to their bodies and progress at their own pace. This approach ensures that everyone feels welcomed and valued, significantly enhancing their learning experience.

Understanding the unique requirements of chair yoga students is key. Many may be dealing with mobility issues, chronic pain, or other health challenges, making traditional yoga poses inaccessible. Your role involves creatively adapting these poses to suit seated positions, ensuring that every student can participate and benefit from the practice.

Clear communication is the cornerstone of effective teaching. Offer concise instructions and provide explanations for each pose, including its benefits. This not only aids in proper execution but also helps students connect more deeply with their practice. Be open to questions and offer personalized guidance whenever necessary. Listening actively to your students' concerns and feedback will make your teaching more effective and rewarding for both you and them.

Safety should be your top priority. Make sure to demonstrate each pose before having your students perform it, highlighting any potential risks and how to avoid them. It's also essential to be aware of common contraindications related to certain health conditions and to advise students accordingly. Encourage students to seek medical advice if they're unsure whether chair yoga is suitable for them.

Motivation plays a crucial role in keeping your students engaged and dedicated to their practice. Celebrate their progress and milestones, no matter how small they may seem. This can significantly boost their confidence and commitment to chair yoga. Incorporating stories of transformation and testimonials from other chair yogis can also be highly inspiring for your class.

As a teacher, continuing your own education is fundamental. Attend workshops, take additional courses, and stay updated with the latest practices and research in chair yoga. This commitment to learning will not only enrich your knowledge but also ensure that your teaching methods remain fresh, relevant, and effective.

Creating a community among your students can be incredibly beneficial. Encourage interactions and discussions before or after class sessions, fostering a support network where everyone feels comfortable sharing experiences, challenges, and achievements. This sense of belonging can greatly enhance the holistic benefits of chair yoga.

Integrating breathing techniques and meditation into your practice is another essential aspect of chair yoga. Teach your students the power of the breath in enhancing physical and mental well-being. Guided meditations can help promote relaxation and stress relief, making the practice more comprehensive and therapeutic.

Incorporating props into your classes can add variety and accommodate different abilities. Items like belts, blocks, and even simple household objects can make poses more accessible or challenging, catering to a wider range of students. Demonstrating how to use these props effectively can greatly enhance the practice.

Adaptability is a must-have trait for any chair yoga teacher. Be prepared to modify your planned sequences based on the day's attendance, noting the specific needs and energy levels of your class. This flexibility ensures that your sessions remain responsive to and appropriate for your students on any given day.

Emphasize the importance of consistency in practice. Encourage your students to integrate chair yoga into their daily routine, whether through a full session or just a few poses throughout the day. This consistent practice can lead to significant improvements in health and well-being over time.

Lastly, remember to practice self-care. Teaching, especially within the realm of chair yoga, can be emotionally and physically demanding. Taking time for your own practice, relaxation, and professional development is crucial in maintaining your energy and passion for teaching.

Being a chair yoga teacher offers a unique opportunity to make a profound impact on the lives of others. By following these guidelines, you can ensure that your teaching not only fosters physical health and flexibility but also cultivates mental and emotional well-being. Embrace this journey with an open heart and mind, and watch as both you and your students flourish.

Adapting Practices for Different Audiences

When guiding others in the rejuvenating path of chair yoga, a one-size-fits-all approach doesn't suffice. People come from diverse backgrounds, with unique physical abilities and health goals. It's crucial, as a teacher, to meet them where they're at, tailor your practice to their needs, and help them discover the joy and benefits of yoga. Let's delve into how you can adapt chair yoga practices for different audiences, ensuring a fulfilling and accessible yoga journey for everyone.

Firstly, understanding your audience is the cornerstone of an effective chair yoga session. Are you teaching seniors seeking to maintain their flexibility and balance? Or perhaps office workers looking for stress relief and a midday energy boost? Maybe you're working with individuals recovering from injuries or with limited mobility. Each of these groups has distinct needs and capabilities, demanding modifications both in the poses offered and the language used to instruct them.

For seniors, it's imperative to focus on safety and the prevention of injuries. Emphasize gentle stretches, balance poses, and movements that enhance flexibility. Utilize props liberally to offer support and make poses more accessible. Remember, the primary goal for this demographic is to maintain or improve quality of life, so prioritizing movements that aid in daily activities is key.

In contrast, when teaching office workers, the focus might be more on relieving tension in the back, neck, and shoulders – areas that suffer due to prolonged sitting. Short, energizing sequences that can be done in work attire without sweating can be particularly beneficial. Poses that can be performed discreetly at a desk can also be a game-changer for this group, combating the fatigue that comes from staring at a screen all day.

For individuals with limited mobility or those recovering from injury, adaptation is paramount. This is where your creativity as a teacher comes in. Modifying poses to accommodate physical limitations, using chairs not only for seated poses but also as support for standing poses, and ensuring that transitions between poses are safe and doable for your students are essential considerations. It's also vital to foster an environment where students feel comfortable voicing their needs and limitations.

Amidst all these adjustments, breathing techniques and meditation should remain a constant. These practices are universally beneficial, promoting relaxation, stress relief, and an increased sense of well-being. Adjust the complexity and duration of these practices based on your audience's familiarity and comfort level with meditation and mindfulness exercises.

Language and communication are just as important as the physical practices. Use clear, simple instructions and avoid yoga jargon that might confuse beginners or those not steeped in the yoga tradition. Encourage feedback, and be observant, ready to adapt your instruction based on the response from your students. Positive reinforcement goes a long way in building confidence and creating an inclusive environment.

An integral part of adapting your teaching involves continuous learning and self-reflection. Stay informed about the latest research in yoga practices, especially those pertaining to chair yoga. Attend workshops, connect with other yoga teachers, and collect feedback from your students to refine your methods and approach.

Utilize props not only as aids for performing poses but also as teaching tools. Props can be instrumental in making poses more accessible and in demonstrating variations of a pose. This not only accommodates different physical capabilities but also helps students understand the versatility and adaptability of yoga.

Developing sequences that cater to the specific needs of your audience is another aspect of customization. For instance, sequences for seniors might have a stronger emphasis on balance and joint mobility, while sequences for office workers might prioritize stretching and relieving tension in the upper body.

Motivation and inspiration are key components of teaching. Share success stories of how chair yoga has positively impacted individuals with similar backgrounds or challenges as your students. This not only motivates but also builds a sense of community and collective aspiration among your students.

Finally, consider the physical space and how it can be adapted to suit the needs of your class. Ensure there is ample room for movement, and if possible, arrange the chairs in a circle or semi-circle to foster a sense of community and allow for easier interaction.

In embracing the diversity of your students and adapting your practices to meet their needs, you contribute to the transformative power of yoga. Chair yoga, with its accessibility and versatility, is a powerful tool in this journey. Your role as a teacher in facilitating this journey is both a privilege and a responsibility. It's about guiding each student to discover their path to health and flexibility, and in the process, you too will grow and learn.

Remember, the essence of yoga is unity – bringing together body, mind, and spirit. In adapting your practices for different audiences, you're honoring this essence, ensuring that chair yoga is indeed a practice for everyone. Embrace the challenge, and let it enrich your teaching and your personal yoga journey.

Cultivating a Community of Chair Yogis

As we dive into the heart of teaching chair yoga, it's essential to focus not just on the poses and the breath but on the vibrant community that chair yoga can create. Building a community of chair yogis offers support, motivation, and a shared journey towards health and flexibility. Each student brings their unique story to the mat—or in this case, the chair—transforming the practice from a solitary endeavor into a collective expedition towards wellness.

The first step in cultivating this community is to encourage open communication. Creating an environment where participants feel comfortable sharing their experiences and challenges is crucial. It's not just about instructing; it's about listening. You'll find that as people share, the barriers between instructor and student begin to blur, fostering a sense of unity and belonging.

Implementing group practices can significantly bolster this sense of community. Encourage your students to engage in poses together or work in pairs for certain exercises. This approach not only assists in proper technique and safety but also builds camaraderie among the group. The shared laughter, encouragement, and sometimes even struggle, knit the group closer.

Social media and online platforms also offer a great avenue to extend this community beyond the physical space. Creating a group or page where members can share tips, progress, and words of encouragement keeps the community active and engaged. Remember, the aim is to build a supportive network, a haven where everyone feels valued and heard.

One shouldn't underestimate the power of celebrating achievements, no matter how small. Acknowledging a member's progress publicly within the group can significantly boost morale and motivation. It sends a powerful message: 'Your efforts matter, and they are recognized.' This celebration of milestones cultivates an environment of positivity and encouragement.

Introducing collaborative events, such as charity yoga sessions or wellness workshops, can also enhance the sense of community. Events like these provide an opportunity for chair yogis to interact in a less structured environment, fostering natural connections and friendships among members.

Feedback is another crucial element in this journey. Providing avenues for members to voice their opinions and suggestions about the classes can make them feel like active contributors to the group's evolution. This inclusive approach will not only improve the teaching quality but also strengthen the community, making members feel like they have a stake in it.

Encouraging mindfulness and presence within the group setting promotes a shared spiritual journey. Integrating guided meditations focusing on gratitude and interconnectedness can deepen these bonds, creating a collective appreciation for the present moment and for each other.

It's also beneficial to share stories of transformation within the group. Whether it's a physical improvement, a mental shift, or an emotional breakthrough, sharing these narratives can be incredibly inspiring. It reminds members why they started and highlights the profound impact chair yoga can have on their lives.

However, while cultivating this community, it's crucial to maintain respect for each individual's boundaries and personal space. Not everyone will feel comfortable sharing or participating in group activities, and that's okay. The goal is to offer opportunities for connection, not enforce it. Recognize and honor each person's journey and pace.

Another aspect to consider is diversity and inclusivity. Strive to make your chair yoga community welcoming to all, regardless of age, mobility, ethnicity, or fitness level. Chair yoga's beauty lies in its accessibility, and your community should reflect that inclusivity. This approach not only enriches the group but also aligns with the broader philosophy of yoga.

Finally, it's about patience and persistence. Communities, like gardens, take time to grow. They require nurturing, attention, and care. There will be challenges along the way, but each hurdle is an opportunity to learn and to strengthen the bonds within the group.

By focusing on these aspects, you can cultivate a thriving community of chair yogis. It's about creating a space where each individual can embark on their health and wellness journey, supported by the collective energy and compassion of the group. Remember, at its core, yoga is about connection—connection to oneself, to others, and to the world around us. Through chair yoga, you are not just teaching movements; you're nurturing a community that uplifts and sustains its members on their paths to health and flexibility.

Teaching chair yoga, therefore, transcends the physical aspects of the practice. It's about guiding individuals to find strength, flexibility, and peace not only in their bodies but in their hearts and minds. As a teacher, you have the unique opportunity to weave a tapestry of diverse threads into a vibrant and supportive community, one chair yogi at a time.

In conclusion, the journey of cultivating a community of chair yogis is both rewarding and transformative. It enriches the teaching experience and provides a profound, shared path to wellness. Through dedication, understanding, and empathy, you can create a space where everyone belongs and thrives. Together, you'll discover that the true power of chair yoga lies in the communal pursuit of health, flexibility, and, ultimately, a fulfilled life.

Chapter 13:
The Future of Chair Yoga

As we delve into the future of Chair Yoga, it's essential to recognize the powerful trajectory this form of exercise is on, evolving to meet the needs of an increasingly diverse population seeking health, flexibility, and peace of mind. The innovation within Chair Yoga practices is rapidly expanding, making it an accessible form of wellness that transcends age, ability, and lifestyle. The foundation of Chair Yoga stands firm on accessibility, but as we look ahead, it's gearing up to integrate cutting-edge approaches that harness technology and community building, ensuring it remains relevant and beneficial for generations to come. The journey toward building an inclusive Chair Yoga movement is not just a vision but a necessary evolution. This movement aims to dismantle barriers, creating a global community where health and wellness are not privileges but innate rights accessible to all. As you embrace Chair Yoga, you're not just adopting a practice for today; you're pioneering a healthier future for everyone, proving that transformation and wellness are within everyone's reach. The future of Chair Yoga is a promise of growth, inclusivity, and boundless potential—embrace it as your pathway to a life well-lived, filled with vitality, strength, and serenity.

Innovations in Chair Yoga Practices

As we move forward into the future, the evolution of chair yoga stands as a beacon of hope and innovation for bringing health and wellness into the lives of many. The continuous growth and adaptation in chair yoga practices ensure that this form of exercise remains accessible, enjoyable, and, most importantly, effective. With creativity and inclusivity at its core, chair yoga is set to break new grounds, making wellness a reachable goal for everyone, regardless of their physical capabilities.

The integration of technology in chair yoga is a significant leap forward. Imagine, if you will, participating in a chair yoga class from the comfort of your home, guided by a virtual instructor who is equipped with AI to personalize your session based on your needs and feedback. This isn't a distant future scenario; it's happening now. These technological advancements make chair yoga not just accessible but highly adaptable to individuals' unique health requirements and preferences.

Digital platforms have made it possible for chair yoga practitioners to connect with others worldwide, fostering a global community of health and wellness supporters. This sense of belonging and connection greatly benefits mental health, providing motivation and encouragement from peers who share similar goals and struggles. Digital classes and apps offer a range of sessions focusing on everything from stress relief to strengthening exercises, ensuring there's something for everyone.

Another notable innovation is the intersection of chair yoga with other holistic practices. Think chair yoga combined with mindfulness meditation or breathing techniques specifically designed to enhance the yoga experience. These combinations offer a more comprehensive approach to wellness, addressing not just physical health but mental and emotional wellbeing too.

Personalization is key in the future of chair yoga. With advancements in wearable technology, practitioners can now track their progress in real-time, receiving feedback on posture, breath, and even heart rate. This information can be used to tailor practices to the individual's day-to-day needs, maximizing the benefits of each session.

For those with specific health conditions, chair yoga is becoming an increasingly important part of treatment plans. Collaborations between healthcare professionals and chair yoga instructors are leading to specialized programs designed for people with conditions like arthritis, diabetes, and chronic pain. These targeted sessions can significantly improve quality of life, providing relief where traditional medicine falls short.

The inclusivity of chair yoga is one of its most appealing features. Adaptive tools and props have evolved, making poses more accessible to individuals with disabilities or limited mobility. From specially designed chairs to supports that aid in maintaining balance and alignment, these innovations ensure everyone can participate and benefit from chair yoga.

Eco-friendly practices are also taking center stage. From the materials used in yoga chairs and props to the digital delivery of classes, reducing the carbon footprint of chair yoga is a priority for many. This commitment to sustainability not only benefits the planet but also aligns with the yogic principle of Ahimsa, or non-harm.

Community-based chair yoga programs have emerged as powerful tools for social change. By offering classes in community centers, schools, and even workplaces, chair yoga is becoming embedded in the daily lives of individuals, promoting health and wellness beyond the traditional studio setting.

Research and education in chair yoga are expanding, with more studies highlighting its benefits and more training programs for instructors. This commitment to understanding and developing chair yoga ensures that practices are both evidence-based and safe, paving the way for future innovation.

At the heart of all these innovations is the desire to make wellness accessible to all. Chair yoga's adaptability and inclusiveness have made it a favorite among many seeking a healthier lifestyle. Its future lies in the community's hands - practitioners, instructors, and innovators alike - who are continually pushing the boundaries of what's possible in the realm of health and wellness.

Finally, the future of chair yoga is not just about new poses or technology; it's about building a movement that prioritizes accessibility, inclusivity, and compassion. As chair yoga continues to evolve, it reaffirms the belief that wellness is a right, not a privilege, and that everyone, no matter their physical condition, has access to a healthier and happier life.

In conclusion, the innovations in chair yoga practices are paving the way for a future where health and wellness are within everyone's reach. With each step forward, chair yoga becomes more integrated into lives, encouraging strength, flexibility, and peace of mind. As we embrace these innovations, we're not just practicing yoga; we're nurturing a global community dedicated to wellness and positivity.

Embrace the innovations in chair yoga and allow them to guide you towards a healthier lifestyle. Remember, your journey to wellness begins with a single step, or in this case, a single pose. Let's make that move together, towards a future where everyone can experience the joy and benefits of chair yoga.

Building an Inclusive Chair Yoga Movement

In the grand tapestry of wellness, chair yoga emerges not just as a practice but as a vibrant movement, steering us toward an inclusive future. As we venture into the heart of inclusivity, let's dive into how chair yoga doesn't just accommodate but wholeheartedly embraces every body and soul, striving to break the barriers of traditional yoga practices.

The genesis of chair yoga was rooted in accessibility, making the profound benefits of yoga available to those who might find traditional forms daunting or unfeasible. This noble foundation paves the way for a broader, more inclusive movement where wellness isn't a privilege; it's a shared right.

Mike Ezekiel

Everyone, regardless of age, mobility, health status, or background, should have access to the transformative powers of yoga.

Imagine a world where wellness spaces radiate with the spirit of inclusivity, where chair yoga classes are as commonplace as any other. In this vision, studios, community centers, and even virtual platforms offer chair yoga, ensuring that these life-enhancing practices are within arm's reach of all who seek them.

To foster an inclusive chair yoga movement, it's imperative we educate and advocate. Education about chair yoga's benefits and potential can demystify practices for skeptics and encourage newcomers. Advocacy for more chair yoga offerings in communal spaces can ignite local changes, catalyzing a ripple effect that spans globally.

Let's not forget the power of community. Building a supportive and welcoming community around chair yoga can amplify its reach and impact. Through social media, local events, and word of mouth, we can spread the word, share experiences, and connect people to this adaptable form of yoga.

Instructors play a pivotal role in this movement. By equipping them with the skills and knowledge to teach chair yoga effectively, we ensure that classes are both empowering and safe. A teacher's enthusiasm and understanding can transform apprehension into confidence, welcoming more people into the fold of yoga practitioners.

Adaptations and modifications of poses are the keystones of chair yoga. They affirm that yoga truly is for every body, underscoring the movement's inclusive ethos. Educating practitioners on how to tailor poses to their needs fosters autonomy and a deeper connection with their practice.

Technology, too, can be a formidable ally in building an inclusive chair yoga movement. Online classes and resources can bridge gaps, making it possible for those in remote or underserved areas to engage with and benefit from chair yoga. Innovation in digital wellness can further personalize and enhance the chair yoga experience for individuals worldwide.

Visibility is crucial. Sharing stories of transformation through chair yoga can inspire others to embark on their journeys of wellness. These narratives not only showcase the transformative power of chair yoga but also reflect the diversity of its practitioners, underscoring the movement's inclusive nature.

Partnerships with healthcare providers can also bolster the movement. When medical professionals recommend chair yoga as part of holistic care plans, it underscores the practice's health benefits and encourages people to incorporate it into their lives for wellness and recovery.

Research plays a significant role as well. By supporting and conducting studies on chair yoga's benefits, we can provide empirical evidence that advocates for its inclusion in wellness programs, insurance packages, and more, further broadening its accessibility and appeal.

Accessibility should also be technological. Ensuring online resources, virtual classes, and digital platforms are user-friendly for people of all ages and abilities can remove barriers to access. Simple, intuitive interfaces and readily available support can make the world of difference.

The inclusive chair yoga movement calls for unwavering commitment to empathy and adaptation. As we forge ahead, let's remember that the heart of chair yoga lies in its adaptability and accessibility. It's a beacon for inclusivity in wellness, illuminating pathways for everyone to embrace yoga's transformative potential.

Finally, the journey toward a more inclusive chair yoga movement is perpetual. It thrives on innovation, compassion, and community. Together, let's envision and work toward a future where chair yoga is unequivocally for all, transcending barriers and uniting us in wellness and flexibility. This isn't just the future of chair yoga; it's the future of a more inclusive and healthier world.

In conclusion, building an inclusive chair yoga movement is more than a goal; it's a journey that we embark on together. It embodies the essence of yoga – union. By welcoming diversity, encouraging adaptability, and fostering community, we're not just practicing yoga; we're living its deepest teachings. Let this be our collective intention as we move forward, embracing every opportunity to make chair yoga an accessible bridge to health and flexibility for every body.

Chapter 14:
Your Journey Toward Health and Flexibility

As we close the final pages of this guide, it's important to reflect on the transformative journey you've embarked upon. Embracing chair yoga isn't just about adopting a new set of exercises; it's about welcoming a profound lifestyle shift that promotes health, flexibility, and wellness. This journey, layered with small, purposeful steps, has the potential to guide you toward a more vibrant version of yourself.

Remember, every individual's path to wellness is unique. The strategies, exercises, and insights shared throughout this book are designed to empower you with knowledge and tools. But the true magic happens when you apply these with consistency, patience, and compassion towards yourself. Health and flexibility, both physical and mental, are not destinations but processes that evolve with you.

Engaging in chair yoga is a testament to the commitment you've made to nurture your body and mind. It's an act of self-love that quietly, yet powerfully, transforms your being. The flexibility we speak of doesn't just apply to the ability to touch your toes but extends to a flexible mindset that welcomes growth, resilience, and positivity.

Mike Ezekiel

Throughout your practice, you may encounter days filled with motivation and others where the couch seems more appealing. This is natural. What's important is showing up for yourself, even if it means just breathing deeply for five minutes or doing a single pose. Celebrating these small victories ignites a fire that fuels your journey forward.

Integration of chair yoga into your daily life, as discussed, can take many forms. Maybe it's a morning routine that greets the day with intention, or perhaps it's those five-minute stretches that break up your workday, bringing renewed energy and focus. Your routine doesn't have to be perfect; it just has to work for you, enhancing your life and wellbeing.

It's also crucial to embrace the holistic approach chair yoga offers. The connection between movement, breath, and mindfulness is a powerful trinity that serves as the cornerstone of your practice. It teaches you to live in the moment, to listen to your body's needs, and to find peace amidst chaos—a skill that transcends the mat and enriches every facet of your life.

Fuel your body with the nutrition it deserves. The principles of mindful eating and the nutritional guidance provided are not about restrictive diets but nurturing your body with what it needs to thrive. Just like a plant needs sunlight, water, and soil, your body requires a balance of nutrients to support your yoga practice and overall wellness.

Let the stories of transformation inspire you but also remind you that progress is deeply personal. Comparisons can be thieving of joy. Measure your success by the milestones you've overcome, not by looking at someone else's journey.

Every body and every life is different; honor yours with kindness and patience.

For those inspired to share the gift of chair yoga, teaching is a pathway that not only enhances your understanding but enriches your soul. The guidelines provided are a foundation from which you can grow, innovate, and inspire others. Community is at the heart of chair yoga, and by fostering it, you contribute to a movement that uplifts and supports.

The future of chair yoga brims with potential. As a dynamic and adaptive practice, it's ever-evolving to meet the needs and challenges of its practitioners. Staying informed, curious, and innovative ensures that your practice grows with you, offering nourishment and challenge in equal measure.

As you continue on this journey, remember that setbacks are not failures but opportunities for growth. Flexibility in practice means adapting without judgment, learning from feedback, and evolving strategies as you progress. It's about finding the balance between effort and ease, pushing boundaries while respecting limits.

Keep nourishing your practice with regular reflection, education, and connection with the chair yoga community. The stories you share, the challenges you overcome, and the insights you gain become part of a larger narrative that shapes the future of this inclusive and transformative practice.

In closing, your journey toward health and flexibility, enriched by chair yoga, is a beacon of light in your life. It illuminates the importance of caring for oneself, embracing change, and facing life's challenges with a grounded and resilient spirit. This journey, unique and beautiful, is yours to continue, with each day offering a new opportunity for growth, discovery, and wellness.

As the pages of this book end, your journey doesn't. Let the practice of chair yoga be a lifelong companion, a source of strength and joy, guiding you toward a life lived with intention, health, and harmony. Here's to your health, flexibility, and the many victories—big and small—waiting on your path ahead. Embrace them with an open heart and mind.

Appendix

Navigating the waters of a healthier lifestyle can be both exhilarating and daunting. As we conclude this guide, remember that every journey begins with a single step—or in this case, a single pose. This appendix is designed to arm you with additional support as you venture into the enriching world of Chair Yoga. Here, you'll find resources and answers to commonly asked questions, serving as your compass along this transformative path.

Recommended Resources for Further Learning

Extending your knowledge and practice beyond what's covered in this book is crucial for growth. Here are some hand-picked resources that can illuminate your path:

Online Communities: Platforms like Yoga Forums and Reddit's r/yoga provide vibrant communities where practitioners at all levels share experiences, advice, and encouragement.

Books: "The Heart of Chair Yoga" by Karen O'Donnell Clarke offers deep dives into the philosophy behind the poses and how to adapt them to your needs.

Videos: YouTube channels like Yoga With Adriene cater to yoga practitioners of all levels, with some content specifically dedicated to Chair Yoga.

Apps: Apps such as Down Dog and Yoga Studio offer customizable yoga practices, including Chair Yoga options, tailored to your preferences and goals.

Common FAQs About Chair Yoga

Can Chair Yoga help with weight loss? While Chair Yoga is a low-impact form of exercise that primarily focuses on flexibility, balance, and strength, it can be part of a holistic approach to weight loss that also includes proper nutrition and mindfulness.

How often should I practice Chair Yoga to see improvements? Consistency is key. Aim for at least two to three sessions a week, but remember, even a few minutes a day can make a difference over time.

Is Chair Yoga safe for those with chronic health conditions? Yes, Chair Yoga can be incredibly beneficial and safe for individuals with chronic conditions. However, consulting with a healthcare provider before starting any new exercise program is always recommended.

Do I need any special equipment? A sturdy chair without wheels is the primary necessity. Beyond that, props like yoga blocks or a strap can be helpful but are not mandatory. You can often use items found around the house as substitutes.

Embracing a healthier lifestyle through Chair Yoga is a journey of self-discovery, resilience, and empowerment. As you explore the vast ocean of resources and tailor your practice to fit your unique needs, remember that every pose, every breath, and every moment of mindfulness brings you one step closer to the vibrant health and vitality you seek. Let your practice be a lighthouse guiding you through the highs and lows, illuminating your path toward wellness. Here's to the journey ahead—may it be enlightening, enriching, and full of growth.

Recommended Resources for Further Learning

Embarking on the journey toward a healthier lifestyle through chair yoga is a commendable decision. It's a path that not only enhances physical flexibility and strength but also nurtures the mind and spirit. To support you on this transformative journey, we've curated a list of resources that will deepen your understanding, inspire your practice, and connect you with a community of like-minded individuals. Let's dive into these treasures that await your exploration.

Books and Guides: Begin with comprehensive books specifically focused on chair yoga. These texts provide a strong foundation, offering detailed pose descriptions, the science behind the practices, and sequences for varied needs. "Chair Yoga: Seated Exercises for Health and Wellbeing" by Edelstein is a great start. It balances instructional content with inspirational stories, showcasing how chair yoga is accessible and beneficial for everyone.

Online Courses and Videos: In our digital age, online platforms are invaluable for learning and practice. Websites like YogaJournal and Gaia offer video tutorials ranging from beginner to advanced chair yoga sequences. These visual guides are perfect for refining your technique and keeping your practice fresh and engaging.

Podcasts and Interviews: Listening to chair yoga practitioners and teachers share their experiences can be incredibly motivating. Podcasts such as "The Yoga Podcast" frequently feature episodes dedicated to chair yoga, covering everything from personal transformation stories to practical tips for incorporating yoga into daily life.

Local Workshops and Retreats: Immersing yourself in a community of chair yogis through workshops and retreats can exponentially enhance your practice. It's an opportunity to learn from experienced instructors, ask questions, and connect with others on similar paths. Look for events in your area that cater to all experience levels.

Academic Research and Articles: For those interested in the scientific underpinnings of chair yoga, academic journals and health publications are treasure troves of information. Research studies demonstrate the physical, mental, and emotional benefits of chair yoga, providing a deeper understanding and validation of your practice.

Yoga Accessories and Props Suppliers: Utilizing props can greatly enhance your chair yoga experience. Look for suppliers that specialize in yoga gear, offering products such as blocks, straps, and cushions. Quality props can aid in alignment, deepen stretches, and increase accessibility of various poses.

Nutrition and Wellness Resources: Integrating mindful eating and wellness habits alongside your chair yoga practice amplifies the benefits. Resources focusing on nutrition, especially those which align with yoga principles, can guide you towards making dietary choices that support your overall well-being.

Community Forums and Social Media Groups: Engaging with an online community through forums and social media can provide support, answer questions, and offer a platform for sharing successes and challenges. Platforms like Reddit and Facebook have active chair yoga groups where members share advice, experiences, and encouragement.

Mindfulness and Meditation Apps: Complementing your chair yoga practice with mindfulness and meditation amplifies its benefits. Apps such as Headspace and Calm offer guided meditations, breathing exercises, and mindfulness challenges that enhance mental clarity and emotional resilience.

Fitness Trackers and Wellness Apps: To monitor your progress and stay motivated, consider using fitness trackers and wellness apps that offer features specifically for yogis. Many apps allow you to set goals, track your practices, and even remind you to stay hydrated and mindful throughout the day.

Subscription-Based Yoga Services: For a more structured and diverse practice, subscription-based services provide access to a vast library of yoga classes, including chair yoga. These platforms often feature world-renowned instructors and offer the flexibility of practicing anytime, anywhere.

Yoga Conferences and Expos: Attending yoga conferences and expos can be enlightening for chair yogis. These events showcase the latest trends, research, and products in the yoga world. They also offer workshops and classes taught by leading yoga practitioners, providing a unique opportunity for learning and networking.

Inspirational Biographies and Memoirs: Sometimes, the most powerful motivation comes from reading about others' journeys. Biographies and memoirs of yogis offer insight into the transformative power of yoga practices, including chair yoga. These stories inspire perseverance, passion, and the pursuit of wellness.

As you continue your journey with chair yoga, remember that learning is a never-ending path. Embrace these resources with an open heart and mind. They will not only guide you but also inspire you to discover the fullest expression of your well-being. Together, let's continue to explore, learn, and grow on this journey to a healthier, more vibrant life.

Common FAQs About Chair Yoga

Embarking on a journey through chair yoga is more than just learning new poses; it's adopting a lifestyle that embraces flexibility, well-being, and mental clarity. As you dive into this transformative practice, many questions might arise. Let's address some of the most common queries to ensure your journey is both enlightening and empowering.

What is chair yoga exactly? At its core, chair yoga is a form of yoga that modifies traditional yoga poses so they can be done while seated or using a chair for support. This makes yoga accessible to people who have difficulty standing for long periods or who are confined to sitting due to physical constraints. It's a fantastic way to enjoy the mental and physical benefits of yoga without the stress on joints and muscles.

Can chair yoga really improve my health? Absolutely. Chair yoga offers a plethora of health benefits, including improved flexibility, better concentration, increased strength, and reduced stress levels. Also, it can aid in managing symptoms related to chronic conditions such as arthritis, diabetes, and hypertension. The beauty of chair yoga lies in its adaptability to cater to a wide range of fitness levels and health conditions.

Is chair yoga suitable for beginners? Yes, chair yoga is exceptionally well-suited for beginners. It provides a gentle introduction to the principles and poses of yoga without the intimidation factor that might come with traditional yoga classes. Chair yoga allows you to learn at your own pace, making it a less daunting entry point into the world of yoga.

How often should I practice chair yoga? The frequency of your practice depends on your individual goals and schedule. However, incorporating chair yoga into your routine several times a week can significantly impact your physical and mental well-being. Even just a few minutes a day can be beneficial. Listen to your body and adjust your practice as needed.

Do I need special equipment for chair yoga? One of the great things about chair yoga is its minimal need for equipment. A sturdy, armless chair is often all you need to get started. As you progress, you might find that props like yoga straps or blocks can help deepen your practice, but these are not required to begin.

Can chair yoga help with stress? Indeed, one of the most celebrated benefits of chair yoga is its ability to reduce stress and promote relaxation. The focus on mindful breathing and gentle stretching helps calm the mind, alleviate anxiety, and enhance overall mood. It's an accessible way to incorporate stress management techniques into your daily life.

What if I have limited mobility? Chair yoga is particularly beneficial for those with limited mobility. It offers a safe and effective way to improve strength, flexibility, and balance without the risk of strain or injury. Always consult with a healthcare provider before beginning any new exercise regimen, and work with a qualified instructor who can adapt poses to meet your needs.

Will chair yoga help me lose weight? While chair yoga is more gentle than some other forms of exercise, it can still contribute to weight loss by increasing muscle tone, improving metabolism, and enhancing digestive health. Paired with a balanced diet and healthy lifestyle choices, chair yoga can be a part of a comprehensive weight management plan.

How does chair yoga differ from traditional yoga? The primary difference is the use of a chair either as the main support for exercises or as an aid for standing poses. This modification makes yoga poses more accessible while still offering the core benefits of traditional yoga, such as increased flexibility, strength, and mental clarity.

Can chair yoga improve my balance? Yes, many chair yoga poses focus on improving core strength and stability, which are essential components of balance. Gradually, as you continue with your practice, you might notice an enhanced ability to maintain poses and a greater sense of physical confidence.

What should I wear for chair yoga? Comfort is key. Opt for loose-fitting or stretchy clothing that allows for a full range of motion. You'll be stretching and bending, so make sure your clothes don't restrict your movement. Shoes are generally not required since many practices are done while seated.

How can I find a chair yoga class? Many yoga studios and community centers now offer chair yoga classes. There's also a wealth of online resources, including video tutorials and virtual classes, allowing you to practice in the comfort of your own home. Remember to look for programs tailored to your fitness level and health needs.

Can I practice chair yoga if I'm pregnant? Chair yoga can be a gentle way for pregnant women to stay active, reduce stress, and prepare for labor. However, it's crucial to consult with your healthcare provider beforehand and work with an instructor experienced in prenatal yoga to ensure the safety of you and your baby.

Is age a barrier to practicing chair yoga? Absolutely not. Chair yoga is celebrated for its inclusivity, offering a welcoming entry point for individuals of all ages. Whether you're in your 20s or your 80s, chair yoga can be adapted to suit your fitness level and mobility, making it a lifelong practice for many.

Taking the plunge into chair yoga can be a transformative step towards a healthier, more vibrant life. Remember, the journey is your own, and every small step is a victory. Embrace the process, listen to your body, and discover the joy of moving more freely and living more fully.

www.ingramcontent.com/pod-product-compliance
Lightning Source LLC
Chambersburg PA
CBHW020425290526

45785CB00002B/726